Clinical Dysarthria

Clinical Dysarthria

Edited by
William R. Berry, Ph.D.

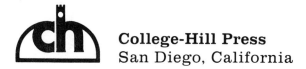

College-Hill Press
San Diego, California

College-Hill Press, Inc.
4580-E Alvarado Canyon Road
San Diego, California 92120

Library of Congress Cataloging in Publication Data

Main entry under title:

Clinical dysarthria.

  "Clinical dysarthria eminated from a conference held in Tucson, AZ., Feb., 10-13th 1982" — CIP pref.
  Bibliography: p.
  Includes index.
  1. Articulation disorders — Congresses. I. Berry, William Robert. [DNLM: 1. Speech disorders — Congresses. WM 475 B5345c 1982]
RC424.7.C57   1982   616.85′5   82-19867

ISBN   0-933014-76-7

Printed in the United States of America

Contents

I

Nature of Dysarthria: Varied Perspectives

II

Assessment and Differential Diagnosis

III

Treatment

Contributors

James H. Abbs, Ph.D.
Speech Motor Control Laboratories
University of Wisconsin
Madison, WI 53706

Beth M. Ansel, M.S.
Department of Communicative Disorders
Speech Motor Control Laboratories
University of Wisconsin
Madison, WI 53706

Richard M. Armour
Speech and Hearing Center
George Washington University
Washington, DC 20052

C. Bruce Baird
Speech and Hearing Center
George Washington University
Washington, DC 20052

James T. Baird, Ph.D.
Speech and Hearing Center
George Washington University
Washington, DC 20052

Steven M. Barlow, M.S.
Speech Motor Control Laboratories
University of Wisconsin
Madison, WI 53706

Gary J. Barnes, M.S.
Department of Audiology and Speech Pathology
Memphis State University
Memphis, TN 38105

Celia J. Bassich, M.A.
Communicative Disorders Program
National Institute of Neurological and
    Communicative Disorders and Stroke
7550 Wisconsin Avenue - Room 1C-13
Bethesda, MD 20205

William R. Berry, Ph.D.
Veterans Administration Medical Center
Memphis, TN 38104

David R. Beukelman, Ph.D.
Department of Rehabilitation Medicine RJ-30
University of Washington
Seattle, WA 98195

Diane M. Bless, Ph.D.
University of Wisconsin
Department of Communicative Disorders
1975 Willow Drive
Madison, WI 53706

Michael P. Caligiuri
Veterans Administration Medical Center
San Diego, CA 92161

Frederic Darley, Ph.D.
Speech Pathology Department
Mayo Clinic
Rochester, MN 55901

Anthony B. De Feo
Department of Speech/Hearing Sciences
University of Arizona
Tucson, AZ 85719

Pamela Enderby, Msc, LCST
Frenchay Hospital
Bristol, England BS1611LE

James Farrage, D.D.S.
Boys Town Institute for Communication
    Disorders in Children
Omaha, NE 68131

Edward L. Goshorn
Veterans Administration Medical Center (126)
1030 Jefferson Avenue
Memphis, TN 38104

Wayne R. Hanson, Ph.D.
Veterans Administration Medical Center (126)
Sepulveda, CA 91343

Chauncey J. Hunker, M.S.
Speech Motor Control Laboratories
University of Wisconsin
Madison, WI 53706

Craig W. Linebaugh, Ph.D.
Speech & Hearing Center
George Washington University
Washington, DC 20052

Roxanne dePaul McNamara, M.S.
Graduate Study
City University of New York
New York, NY

Christy L. Ludlow, Ph.D.
Communicative Disorders Program
National Institute of Neurological and
   and Communicative Disorders and Stroke
7550 Wisconsin Avenue, Room 1C-13
Bethesda, MD 20205

Malcolm R. McNeil, Ph.D.
Department of Communicative Disorders
Speech Motor Control Laboratories
University of Wisconsin
Madison, WI 53706

E. Jeffrey Metter, M.D.
Veterans Administration Medical Center (126)
Sepulveda, CA 91343

Thomas Murry, Ph.D.
Audiology and Speech Pathology Service
Veterans Administration Medical Center
San Diego, CA 92161

Ronald Netsell, Ph.D.
Boys Town Institute for Communication
  Disorders in Children
Omaha, NE 68131

Sara B. Sanders, Ph.D.
Veterans Administration Medical Center
Memphis, TN 38104

Christine Shaefer
Department of Speech/Hearing Sciences
University of Arizona
Tucson, AZ 85719

Ann L. Shaughnessy, M.S.
Boys Town Institute for Communication
  Disorders in Children
Omaha, NE 68131

Nina N. Simmons, M.S.
Louisianna Rehabilitation Institute
1532 Tulane Avenue
New Orleans, LA 70140

Kathryn M. Yorkston, Ph.D.
Department of Rehabilitation Medicine, RJ-30
University of Washington
Seattle, WA 98195

Foreword

Dysarthria appears to have come into its own. Whereas a few years ago one would have been hard put to find a book about it or to find more than cursory allusions to it in speech pathology textbooks, now books and articles abound. And now dysarthria has generated its unique professional meeting—the Clinical Dysarthria Conference, born on February 10, 1982. This publication contains a number of edited presentations from that first conference and demonstrates how far interest in and knowledge about dysarthria have come.

Its beginnings are obscure. It isn't obvious how the word got put together—*arth*- meaning "joint" and *dys*- meaning "abnormal, difficult, faulty, or impaired"—or how exactly one got from the impaired articulation of bones in joints to impaired articulation of phonemes in speech. But the word somehow got made, and for a long time meant "defective articulation of speech." In 1911, Gutzmann pointed out that it is not only articulation that is defective in dysarthria; respiration and voice quality may be disturbed as well as aspects of tempo and pitch. Logically, some have thought that the problem should therefore be called dysarthro-pneumo-phonia, but developments haven't gone *that* far. We pretty well agree today on use of the term dysarthria to refer to a group of speech disorders involving any or all of the basic motor speech processes—respiration, phonation, resonance, articulation, and prosody—resulting from disturbances in muscular control due to damage to the central or peripheral nervous system, always evidenced by some degree of weakness, slowness, incoordination, or alteration of muscle tone of the speech apparatus.

Dysarthria has been a fascinating part of the identification of specific neurologic diseases over the centuries:

• Two hundred and ninety-nine years ago, Willis provided the first description of speech in myasthenia gravis: "She for some time can speak freely and readily enough, but after she has spoke long, or hastily, or eagerly, she is not able to speak a word, but becomes mute as a Fish, nor can she recover the use of her voice under an hour or two."

• In his 1817 "Essay on the Shaking Palsy," Parkinson mentioned his patients' "impediment of speech" and quoted an earlier observer who had reported that the muscles of these patients "with an impetus not to be repressed, accelerate their motion, and run before the unwilling mind."

• We enjoy Lewis Carroll's presentation, in *Alice's Adventures in Wonderland*, of the Mad Hatter with his wild prosody of a familiar song: "Twinkle, twinkle, little bat, how I wonder what you're at." We realize that this 19th century hat maker was sick with a toxic encephalopathy, for he, like his fellows, dipped furs into vats of mercuric nitrate solution to make them pliable, inadvertently absorbing the toxic substance through their skin and inhaling mercury vapor leading to loss of teeth, tremor, gait problems, dementia, and dysarthria.

• In 1877, Charcot described the triad of symptoms of multiple sclerosis —nystagmus, intention tremor, and dysarthria: "The affected person speaks in a slow drawling manner, and sometimes almost unintelligibly... The words are as if measured or scanned; there is a pause after every syllable, and the syllables themselves are pronounced slowly."

• In 1911, Wilson described progressive lenticular degeneration, a disorder now bearing his name, the signs including first "a little slurring," then "definitely impaired articulation," then anarthria, finally speechlessness.

Classification of the disorders embraced by the term dysarthria was first attempted in 1881 by Kussmaul. Variably useful systems later emerged, including that of Grewel in Amsterdam. Monrad-Krohn brought prosody into view as a critical component of dysarthric syndromes. The latest effort to sort out the dysarthrias in terms of their distinctive perceptual phenomenology was that of Aronson, Brown, and Darley, in 1969. Laboratory studies using a variety of instrumental techniques have increasingly been reported and have further clarified the neurophysiology of some of the dysarthrias.

Only in approximately the last 40 years have we seen people with clinical interests begin to cogitate on how to help the dysarthric patient. We recall Samuel D. Robbins' 1940 article in the *Journal of Speech Disorders* on dysarthria and its treatment. In 1951, Baker and Sokoloff offered suggestions on how to help patients with dysarthria resulting from bulbar polio. Froeschels wrote about some of the dysarthrias and produced in 1952 a book, *Dysarthric Speech*, dealing primarily with speech in cerebral palsy. Morley presented articles on the rehabilitation of adults with dysarthric speech in 1955 in the *Journal of Speech and Hearing Disorders*. *Motor Speech Disorders* in 1975 pulled together some ideas of treatment, followed by the Johns-edited *Clinical Management of Neurogenic Communicative Disorders*. Materials are available that summarize and systematize clinical observations and experiences for the guidance of professionals who have awakened to this area of clinical practice.

Now the Clinical Dysarthria Conference has met, and some seventy-five people have spent time together reviewing the state of the art and sharing new insights and new findings. Here we see presented case reports that challenge the limits of our present phenomenological and etiological classifications; analysis of assessment procedures and suggestions for improving measurement; discussion of theoretical issues; and proposals for more effective remediation. This meeting was no mere academic exercise, exploiting a disorder as a vehicle for learning something more about the brain or the linguistic system. It represented a pragmatic approach to a significant patient problem based on the conviction that the most important things we can know about the dysarthrias are how to reduce them and help flesh-and-blood patients cope with them.

Frederic L. Darley

Preface

Clinical Dysarthria emanated from a conference held in Tucson, Arizona, February 10-13, 1982. The chapters included in this volume are a result of invitations to a group of distinguished scientists and clinicians. Portions of these chapters were presented at the Clinical Dysarthria Conference for discussion. The book is divided into three major sections: I) Nature of Dysarthria; II) Assessment and Differential Diagnosis; and III) Treatment.

NATURE OF DYSARTHRIA: VARIED PERSPECTIVES

Abbs, Hunker, and Barlow present a challenging set of data, documenting the motor system breakdown when we evaluate our patients, either diagnostically or serially. Netsell's bolstering presentation elaborates on the remarkable verbal communication system that we must evaluate and treat. Netsell refers to the power of the system to adapt; even though we are analyzing its breakdown. What are the messages of these two highly regarded clinical researchers ? Abbs et al. are calling for more exacting methods to measure the precise point of neuromuscular breakdown; whereas, Netsell reminds us that we must not ignore the functional behavior of the entire system. There must be a balance of the analytic and synthetic approaches.

Barnes continues the first section with a comprehensive review of prosody, a chapter of utmost value to clinicians and scientists. The following chapter by Murry fills a long-felt void in the area of measurement of prosody. Ansel and associates provide a balance of physiological and acoustic approaches to understanding prosody.

ASSESSMENT AND DIFFERENTIAL DIAGNOSIS

Evaluating the individual with dysarthria is a formidable task. The material presented by Netsell, as well as Abbs et al., in Section I makes this glaringly obvious. This section on assessment provides us with practical information and a sense of direction for the evaluation process. Enderby outlines a diagnostic protocol that is based on a functional scale according to the major organ being assessed. The scale provides an innovative tool for the diagnostician to score and interpret motor speech dysfunction.

Ludlow and Bassich, in their chapter, add objectivity to the prevailing assessment techniques by correlating acoustic measures of speech with perceptual judgments. Yorkston and Beukelman present an assessment of intelligibility of dysarthric speech which serves as a model for the treatment of dysarthria via output analysis. The case study by DeFeo and Shaefer is unique in the sense that it outlines a comprehensive multidimensional procedure for treating a dysarthric child with complicating developmental speech and language problems.

TREATMENT

Beginning the discussion on treatment, McNamara, like DeFeo and Shaefer, presents a case illustrating the need for coordinated team intervention in the management of dysarthria. Her case study and the chapter by Berry and Sanders address similar issues, namely, team management. Perhaps the most salient component of the chapters in this section is the overall effectiveness of the patient's communication.

The ensuing five chapters are concerned with individual treatment approaches recommended and implemented by the clinician. Shaughnessy, Netsell, and Farrage describe the combined effects of palatal lift prosthesis with traditional therapy to yield impressive results in the treatment of a 4-year-old with severe velopharyngeal dysfunction. Hanson and Metter review their use of portable delayed auditory feedback (DAF) with patients suffering from Parkinsonism. Berry and Goshorn, as well as Caligiuri and Murry, report single subject designs to test the efficacy of various instrumental feedback techniques. These studies help to illustrate the importance of a clinician-researcher hypothesis. These designs were carefully controlled therapy plans which yielded data where conclusions could be drawn as to the accountability of the therapy protocol. Clinicians may use these reports and implement their treatment for comparable results. In her chapter, Simmons combines an acoustic feedback approach with long-term treatment of a case of ataxic dysarthria.

Linebaugh and his colleagues describe a range of augmentative communication systems in lieu of oral communication. The array of hardware and software now available provides the clinician with yet another facet of intervention and improvement to severely distorted speech neuromotor systems.

All in all, the chapters in these three sections comprehensively address the most compelling and important theoretical, experimental, and clinical aspects of dysarthric speech—all in the context of a clinician. Hence, the title *Clinical Dysarthria.*

This book is dedicated to Frederick L. Darley and to all who might follow his leadership in the treatment of those who suffer from dysarthria.

William R. Berry

Section I

Nature of Dysarthria: Varied Perspectives

1

Speech Motor Control: Theoretical Issues with Clinical Impact

Ronald Netsell

INTRODUCTION

In the past ten to fifteen years, expanded literatures have appeared on (1) the mechanisms of speech motor control in normal and neurologically impaired individuals, and (2) understanding and treating the dysarthrias (see Abbs and Cole, 1982; Hixon, 1982; Netsell, 1982; for reviews). Another literature, dealing with the motor control of other body parts (e.g., the eyes, arms, hands, and legs) in humans and other mammals, is increasing even more rapidly (see Brooks, 1981). In the space available, I have rather presumptuously taken on the task of reviewing some of the current themes and issues of motor control that relate to the dysarthrias. For purposes of this presentation, *speech motor control* is broadly defined as the neuronal actions that initiate and regulate muscle contractions for speech production. The *speech motor system* refers to the neural mechanisms used to produce speech. From the host of topics that could be presented, I have selected ones that most directly influence how I think about speech as a motor skill and how that, in turn, affects my conceptualization of the motor control problem of the dysarthric client under study. Obviously, the questions we ask about "what is going wrong with the speech of this person" are powerfully conditioned by (1) the way we believe normal speech is produced, (2) what goes wrong, from a motor control point of view when given pathways or regions of the nervous system are damaged, and (3) when (in a developmental sense) the damage occurred. It seems likely that most dysarthric movement patterns combine the direct motor control effects of the lesion(s), secondary effects of altered "postural reflexes" (e.g., overall increases or decreases in muscle stiffness), and tertiary effects of intended, or unintended, compensatory adjustments. This raises the question of the extent to which models of normal speech production are applicable to the motor control problems facing dysarthric speakers. This question, along with all others raised in this paper and conference, are basically unanswered. Even though the present answers are fuzzy, the asking of the questions serves several important purposes. First, we squarely face the facts versus fantasies of our current answers. Second, we try to restate the questions in terms of hypotheses for experimental test. Third, we gauge the impact of these questions and answers on each part of our clinical practice.

METRICS OF NORMAL SPEECH

Precision Capabilities

We have the capability to reach highly precise successions of vocal tract shapes, seeming to reach acoustically critical points at critical points in time. That is, we often come within 1 mm of previously attained positions and time the phasing of one articulator movement within 10 msec of another (Kent and Moll, 1975; Netsell, Kent, and Abbs, 1980). These spatial-temporal goals are reached rapidly, interactively (with respect to articulator trade-offs, or "motor equivalence"), and are accomplished automatically (that is, without the conscious awareness of the speaker). This "motor equivalence" is accomplished in the upper airway through automatic velocity and directional changes in the articulator movements (see review in Abbs and Cole, 1982; Netsell et al., 1980. Additional trade-offs are made in the components of the respiratory component for maintaining a constant subglottal air pressure (Hixon, 1982). These adjustments in goal achievement are made in natural speech, in response to small, externally applied loads, or in holding one part of the mechanism in a fixed position. Compared to our fastest movements (for example, those of the eyes), speech is relatively slow, probably using relatively small percentages of the muscles' maximum contractile force and motor units of small-to-intermediate size. Given these metrics, speech production falls into the category of a fine motor skill, similar in principle to playing a piano or violin.

The spatial precision reviewed above only reflects the *capabilities* or limits of the normal speech motor system. This precision may not be used in typical conversation and it can be shown to deteriorate with increases in speaking rate. As will be discussed later, speaking rate is a key variable in evaluating and treating individual dysarthric speakers.

Adaptive Control and Speech Motor Skill[1]

Speech production meets the general requirements of a fine motor skill, viz., it (1) is performed with accuracy and speed, (2) demonstrates motor flexibility in achieving goals, (3) is improved by practice, and (4) relegates all of this to automatic control, where "consciousness" is freed from the details of action plans (Wolff, 1979). As a motor skill, speech is goal-directed and afferent-guided. The goal is to produce the appropriate acoustic patterns via flexible motor *actions* that are formed and maintained by "auditory images." These "auditory images," in turn, become yoked to the motor and somatoafferent patterns used to generate them (see Wolff's discussion of "perceptual motor ideas"). These "ideas" are highly similar to those of others (cf. Bernstein, 1967; Gurfinkel and Levik, 1979; Hardy, 1970; Ladefoged, DeClerk, Lindan, and Papcun, 1972; MacNeilage, 1970).

It is emphasized that these motor *actions* are not fixed movement routines or stored patterns of muscle contractions. The speaker's internal referent is what it "feels" and sounds like to produce certain speech movements and acoustics. Similarly, the "proficient violinist breaks a string while playing a recital but continues the performance without interruption by reprogramming the usual fingering, and playing the required notes on different strings. The 'motor idea' controlling the musical performance does not prescribe a fixed relation between notes and finger movements, but enables the performer to generate functionally equivalent new finger sequences that will all preserve the musical passage" (Wolff, 1979). Comparable skills are evidenced in speech production (see review in Abbs and Cole, in press).

Speech, in requiring adaptive control, represents one of the most advanced examples of selective access to muscles or pattern generators for the purpose of spontaneously creating novel motor acts, i.e., those acts used to express a new thought of the speaker. Although it's reasonable to assume that humans are genetically predisposed to develop speech, they must be exposed to the appropriate sound patterns of a given language and undergo a reasonable period of sensorimotor learning in order to produce these sound patterns.

SPECULATIONS ABOUT NEURONAL MECHANISMS

Phylogeny and Ontogeny

In trying to understand how the human has developed the neuronal mechanisms for speech and language, we can look for clues in the phylogeny and ontogeny of the organism. The concept of the "triune brain" (a reticular to limbic to neocortical progression) is helpful in this regard (Brown, 1979; MacLean, 1970; Mysak, 1976). The current human brain is not viewed as a simple layering-on of new to old brain, but, rather, the elaboration and differentiation of each of the more primitive nervous systems; so that today's human is still very much in touch with, and influenced by, its reticular and limbic systems. Given this view, it's not surprising we have strong subcortical representations of speech, language, and thought. It is difficult to say whether the increased human capabilities are strictly a reflection of quantitative changes, as opposed to qualitative changes, in brain function. Nevertheless, there is little doubt that we possess the highest form of selective access to our motor neurons. This selective access is a key feature to our vocal tract and manual manipulative skills.

In ontogenetic development, myelinization proceeds from the brainstem outward, progressing both to the head and to the feet. Some cortical and subcortical regions develop earlier than others, and each regional development presumably is more complex in terms of the cognitive and sensorimotor functions it mediates. The rates of development even within a given cranial nucleus are differential, and develop to serve the needs of the organism at particular points in time. For example, in the facial nucleus the lower portions develop more rapidly to serve the feeding functions required at birth, whereas the upper regions of this nucleus develop later in innervating the brow and other muscles of facial expression (Anokhin, 1974).

The infant also progresses through stages of "reflex development," where certain primitive and obligatory reflexes gradually disappear in the first six months, and other stereotyped patterns (e.g., righting and equilibrium reactions) appear in the second six months. The persistence of the primitive reflexes may interfere with the development of these reactions and any motor skills that depend on these reactions. It has been suggested that these primitive reflexes are placed under inhibitory control of the cerebrum and that they reappear with cerebral trauma (Capute, Shapiro, Palmer, Accardo, and Wachtel, 1981). A major theoretical issue is whether or not these reflexes or reactions are (1) *incorporated* into skilled motor acts, or (2) *inhibited*, or "gated-out," so as not to interfere with intended movements. Present data are sparse and provide no clear evidence for the incorporated or inhibited hypothesis Capute et al. suggest that of the seven primitive reflexes they have studied, only the tonic labyrinthine significantly affects the oral-motor movements or positioning of normal infants. Obviously, the presence of strong normal or pathologic reflexes in the brain-injured will affect vocal tract movements. This is not to say that these reflexes are part of the speech motor control system.

Distributed Systems and Functions

Another important concept is that of *distributed* systems, especially in the neocortical system (see Mountcastle, 1978).[2] The concept here is that nuclei in different regions of the nervous system form interconnections to serve particular functions. Some functions share particular nuclei and pathways, and not others. In addition, the "command neurons" for the different functions are located at different places in the nervous system. For example, breathing, sucking, chewing, and swallowing are thought to be driven by pacemaker neurons, or "pattern generators," located in the brainstem, whereas human speech motor control depends upon more recently evolved neocortical structures.[3]

The concepts of distributed systems and functions gain some validity from clinical data. For example, selective damage to phylogenetically older parts of the cerebellum may affect walking and not talking. Conversely, walking can be preserved and a severe dysarthria result from damage to the neocerebellum. The distributed concepts also imply it is difficult, if not impossible, to destroy an entire function with a relatively small localized lesion. Likewise, a localized lesion can disturb, at least in part, more than one function. The latter instances are most obvious at "summing points," or "final common pathways," in the nervous system, e.g., at cortical or lower motor neurons where the nerve action potentials for more than one function are transmitted.

And finally, the distributed and distinctive nature of speech and language neural processes can be illustrated through electrical stimulation of different nuclei in the thalamus. Stimulation, even *within* the left ventrolateral nucleus, can either slow down or speed up speech movements (Hessler, 1966; Mateer, 1978), and result in errors in naming or verbal memory (Ojemann and Ward, 1980). Lower stimulation current at these same sites accelerates memory processes, but not speech (Ojemann and Mateer, 1979).

Possible Roles of Afference

In addition to the need for hearing, the develop.nent of normal speech patterns is believed to depend upon *somatoafference*. Somatoafference is defined here as receptor information from the skin, muscles, and joints concerning position and movement.

From afference to action to higher mental functions — Many Russian investigators appear to assign primary importance to afferent mechanisms in developing and controlling skilled actions such as speech. These actions, in turn, are considered essential to the development of "higher mental functions." For example, Luria (1980) says, "In the early stages relatively simple sensory processes, which are the foundation for higher mental functions, play a decisive role; during subsequent stages, when the higher mental functions are being formed, this leading role passes to the more complex systems of connections that develop on the basis of speech, and these systems begin to determine the whole structure of the higher mental processes. For this reason, disturbance of the relatively elementary processes of sensory analysis and integration, necessary, for example, for the further development of speech, will be decisively important in early childhood, for it will cause the underdevelopment of all the functional formations for which it serves as a foundation" (Luria, 1980, p. 35 italics mine). Vygotsky formulated the following rule concerning the influence of a localized lesion at different stages of the development of a function: "In the early stages of ontogenesis, a lesion of a particular area of the cerebral cortex will predominantly affect a higher (that is developmentally dependent upon it) center than that where the lesion is situated, whereas in the stage of a fully formed functional system, a lesion of the same area of the cortex will predominantly affect a lower center (that is regulated by it)" (Luria, 1980, p. 35). Given the earlier discussion of the triune brain and its ontogenetic development, Vygotsky's rule should apply to the *distributed* speech motor system (i.e., brainstem and subcortical systems) as well.

Afferent construction of motor acts — Grillner (1982) speculates that information from any relevant receptor system that is available may be utilized *at the time* a movement is planned to "construct" the motor command to be issued, so as to achieve an optimal pattern of activity. That is, the somatoafference is used by the child in constructing the original individual motor acts and in constructing a sequence of learned motor acts when expressing a novel thought through the speech motor system.

Grillner suggests that once speech motor acts have been learned, they are driven by "central programs," and these central programs use positive feedback as a means to construct the final motor output. This represents "a learned but subconscious type of pattern recognition of afferent information used to guide a central program" (Grillner, 1982, p. 221). With this concept, there is essentially instantaneous appraisal of the motor neurons generating the muscle forces concerning the state of the vocal tract. Earlier concerns that nervous system delays were too long for such fast modulations of motor neuron activity have been lessened by more recent theory and data (Abbs and Cole, 1982; Cole, 1981). Indeed, the neocortical system anatomy is such that both the cerebral and cerebellar cortices can be used in this afferent-efferent process.

Forward-looking control—Most of the concepts of feed forward and forward-looking control systems include some representation of the external world in the brain. For speech, some have suggested we develop a referent in terms of a vocal tract analog (see review in Kent and Minifie, 1977). "If one accepts that the nervous system is probably developed so as to best do the job, then some ahead of time representation of movements is certainly expected" (Rack, 1981, p. 254). There may also be a provisional or initial command ("corollary discharge," "efference copy") that (1) accounts for the peripheral state of the vocal tract (position, velocity, plus perhaps, acceleration), and (2) makes online changes in its controlling signal to the muscles. This internal revision of the controlling signal depends upon past experience as well as the present state of the vocal tract.

The embodiment of "past experience" is most often assigned to another construct of motor learning, viz., the "schema" (plural, "schemata").[4] In terms of speech motor control, schemata can be conceptualized as brain representations of what it "sounds and feels like" to say or think a particular word or sentence.

Levels of Command Specificity

A key theoretical issue in motor control concerns the extent of detail that is specified at the input of the motor system under study. The range of possibilities includes the following: (1) Relative *gross* excitatory and/or inhibitory signals are hypothesized to activate subsequent mechanisms (for example, "neural oscillators" or "pattern generators") which, in turn, carry out quasi-stereotyped motor actions. This option requires minimal detail from the central "motor commands." The detail is in "phasing" the cycles of the "lower level" oscillators, but how this phasing is learned, directed, or regulated for purposes of speech is not well formulated in the current explanations of the theory (see review in Kelso, 1981). (2) An intermediate level of command, or input specificity, calls for more *selective* activation of lower level mechanisms (for example, "pattern generators"), where the neural circuits used (for example, for walking) can be accessed at different points to yield independent movements (for example, flexing only the ankle or toe) (cf. Grillner, 1982). (3) At the level of extreme command specificity is the *direct-line* hypothesis, where the cortical motor neurons have private and rather direct access to the lower motor neurons. This latter view regards cortical motor neurons as a summing point of (1) afferent and efferent information for the control of the muscles, and (2) the words selected to express the speaker's ideas. The essential problem to be solved is the most direct transform possible of the intended thought onto the controlling motor neurons. The controlling neurons have essentially instantaneous information about the present state and/or immediate future state of the vocal tract. This may be sufficient updated and predictive information with which to modulate, *de novo*, the cortical motor neurons. This obviates the need for a provisional command to be revised and allows the "on-line" flexibility to begin vocalizing the thought and continue word selection even before the thought is complete (see Fry, 1966). It is also possible that this creative, "thoughtful" mode of talking engages brain mechanisms different from those used in rote speech, imitation, or repeating nonsense syllables. The direct-line hypothesis relies minimally, if at all, on phylogenetically older mechanisms (e.g., brainstem pattern generators, or neural oscillators). For example, many dysarthric speech patterns are immediately free of disorder with the remission of tremor. It seems as if the neural oscillators have superimposed a pathologic amplitude on otherwise normal speech movements. Once the amplitudes of these oscillations are reduced, the speech is perceived as normal. These clinical observations do not seem compatible with notions of *phasing* or *selectively activating* pattern generators or neural oscillators.

Each of the above hypotheses emphasizes the availability and value of afferent information. None of these hypotheses has represented speech acts as a stringing together of "overlearned, stereotypic" motor patterns. However, the speech motor acts of a given language, once learned, are not infinitely flexible, but quasi-fixed, in that certain tightly coordinated movements cannot be broken up (except by neurologic lesion), and others are extremely difficult to learn or unlearn beyond a certain age.

Given its current sophistication, the human nervous system probably selects the best of its old and new mechanisms to formulate, initiate, and control speech motor acts.

A Continuum of Actions and Modes of Control

It has been suggested that *slow* movements can use limited servo assistance (e.g., via "stretch reflexes"), whereas rapid movements cannot (Rack, 1981). "For *rapid* movements the patterns of motor neuron activity must be computed and sent out without the benefit of immediate information about their effects" (Rack, p. 252). We speculated earlier that speech movements may be of moderate speed and thus benefit from a variety of modes of control. It may also be that different phases of speech movements are differentially controlled, and the same speech pattern (produced at faster speeds) may require shifts in the mode of control. Answers to some of these questions may come when discharge patterns of multiple motor units are studied for a variety of motor acts produced at varying speeds (e.g., comparing labial single motor units during three motor actions, viz., nonspeech movements, saying "papapapapapa," and saying "Buy Bobby a puppy," where each action is produced at slow, intermediate, and fast speeds). An experiment of similar principle has been proposed, where nerve cell recordings at different loci within the monkey's nervous system would be compared for the activities of rhythmical chewing and controlled biting (Luschei and Goldberg, 1981). Burke's (1981) review of motor unit research provides some preliminary evidence that motor neurons are selectively activated for motor actions that are qualitatively different, i.e., under a different mode of control. Patterns of motor neuron recruitment may also differ as a function of speed of movement. Obviously, we'd like answers to questions raised by these issues in considering what types of movements we ask dysarthric clients to make and what we conclude about their motor responses to our requests.

The nature of skilled action patterns—A final issue concerns the assumptions we make about the nature of skilled action patterns, in general, and speech motor actions, in particular. *If* there are encoding "units" smaller than words, what is their size and how, morphologically, are they represented ? Grillner, for example, speculates that speech motor actions are made up of "motor acts," where "each motor act corresponds to a critical configuration of the oral cavity" (in press).

The Question of Unit Size — The available data offer little resolution to the question of "unit size" (see reviews in Kent and Minifie, 1977; MacNeilage, 1970). There are no data to show they are of the size often practiced in speech therapy, i.e., the phone (or phoneme), the consonant-vowel syllable, or other syllable forms. Also, in fractionating words or nonsense syllables into smaller, but potentially artificial, motor acts (e.g., in asking the client to first learn the motor act for *s*, then *ou,* and then *p*), we may be asking the client to learn separate motor acts that are not added together as they would be normally in saying the word "soup." Ideally, we would require practice of the requisite motor acts according to their true size as inputs to the speech motor systems. It also may be that the "size" of these input units changes during the acquisition of the language, although the *word* is an attractive candidate regardless of speaker age.

RELEVANCE TO THE DYSARTHRIAS

It is not possible in the space available to discuss in detail all the ramifications of the foregoing for the clinical matters of the dysarthrias. As with many of the points covered in the previous sections, many of these clinical implications are clearly beyond the data. As such, they are hypotheses to be tested.

Evaluating Speech Neural Mechanisms

Speech versus nonspeech acts—Hixon and Hardy (1964) hypothesized that the most appropriate test of speech neural mechanisms was to observe vocal tract movements during the production of speech. The lumping of all vocal tract movements other than speech into the "nonspeech" category represents a semantic and conceptual hazard. The neuronal machinery and/or patterns of activation responsible for sucking, chewing, swallowing, blowing, imitating orofacial movements, rapid alternating movements (with or without sound production), and isometric muscle contracts are hypothesized to be different from those used for speaking (see Dubner, Sessle, and Storey, 1978; Netsell, 1980). The nonspeech behaviors are often useful in determining the lesion(s) locus and general pathophysiologic consequence, but the activation of the speech neural mechanisms with *meaningful speech* may be the only valid test of function for the speech motor system.

There also is the concern that testing speech motor functions with sustained phonations, nonsense syllables, or "diadochokinesic rates" will yield results different from those gained with linguistically meaningful stimuli. For example, we saw a young boy recently who had substantial velopharyngeal opening when repeating /papapapapa/, but who achieved normal closure for words such as *puppy, papa,* and *puffy.* It is a common clinical observation that velopharyngeal function during a sustained *ah* sound does not predict function during speech for the dysarthria individual. Miller and Hardy (1962) have shown marked differences in motor control of the tongue for speech and nonspeech movements in children with cerebral palsy. Even in normal speakers, laryngeal airflow during sustained vowels is generally lower than in consonant-vowel syllables (Smitheran and Hixon, 1981) and laryngeal resistance to airflow during nonsense syllables can be dramatically different from that recorded during meaningful words (Shaughnessy, Lotz, and Netsell, 1981).

Testing component functions and adaptive control—The value of testing individual components of the speech mechanism is well known (cf. Abbs, this volume; Hardy, 1967; Hixon, 1982; McNamara, this volume; Mysak, 1976; Netsell, 1976; Rosenbek and LaPointe, 1978). For an example, holding the jaw in a fixed position, with a bite-block held between the teeth, is used to test independent functions of the lips and tongue. Better speech performance with the jaw fixed suggests that jaw abnormalities are contributing to the poor speech. Poorer speech with the jaw stablized suggests the jaw is assisting (compensating for) the tongue and/or lips, or, biting on the block results in a spread of hyperactivity to the tongue and/or lips and affects their movements. Poorer performance with the jaw fixed also may indicate that the client has lost the adaptive control discussed earlier as "motor equivalence."

An additional caution in interpreting component functions of the speech mechanism is that they may appear reasonably good on a component-by-component basis but look and sound quite poor collectively. Among the many possible reasons for this would be that the component analysis does not test the overall coordination of the speech mechanism. That is, in fractionating function of the whole system we have failed to test the coordination of the whole system. This concern is lessened by using meaningful speech stimuli that place primary demands on one component and minimal requirements on the others. For example, in testing lip function, use of the words "mom" or "mama" places emphasis on lip movements and lesser demands on the velopharynx, tongue, larynx, and respiratory system. A second reason for collective failure, or poor speech, with reasonably good individual components, is that their summed small deficiencies added to a poor overall function. We recently saw a young man who had mild to moderate involvement of all components, no one of which would account for his generally unintelligible speech. A third hazard is that some components may appear severely involved in the presence of fairly adequate speech. Remaining adaptive control may be compensating for these more severe malfunctions, and treatment of them may be ill-advised. Many dysarthric clients have made adaptations to component malfunctions before coming to the clinic. The clinician must determine if these compensations are maladaptive. If so, they should be rehabilitated with regard to the pattern of deficits in the other components. If the compensations are not maladaptive and yield intelligible speech, the clinician may want to reinforce them and alter speaking rate and/or effort to further increase intelligibility.

Implications for Treatment

Several of the issues raised above bear directly on management decisions for the individual dysarthric client. Treatment considerations are outlined below for (1) restoring functions or skills that were acquired premorbidly, and (2) facilitating speech motor development in the brain-injured child. In general, the treatment approaches are conservative and eclectic. Since we lack data on the effectiveness of most individual and collective treatments, we can only intuit the appropriateness of a given procedure based upon our knowledge of normal and abnormal mechanisms and clinical experience.

Restoration of the speech motor system—In cases of adult dysarthria, the two general goals are to (1) maximize the functional integrity of the musculoskeletal system, i.e., the vocal tract, and (2) require the nervous system to selectively engage its speech motor system.

Methods to optimize the expression of the speech motor system include (1) posturing to minimize the influence of pathologic reflexes (cf. Mysak, 1980); (2) other musculoskeletal alterations such as surgery, palatal lifts, bite-blocks, and abdominal binding; (3) orofacial stimulation and passive range of motion exercises to maintain sensorimotor and neuromuscular integrity, respectively; and (4) *minimal* strengthening exercises to maintain muscle mass. The methods under (3) and (4) are hypothesized to be of little value once some minimal speech movements can be elicited from the vocal tract component of interest. If the client can chew and swallow, this is probably sufficient activity to maintain at least muscle, nerve-muscle, and sensorimotor integrities for the neural mechanisms implicated in (3) and (4) above.

Several principles guide the selection of speech materials to be practiced. The starting points are taken from the client's available speech movements. Words are selected to preferentially activate muscles and muscle synergies over which the client has some control. Phonetic environments are chosen to facilitate the target movements. For example, work with nasal consonants in words could begin even if a substantial velopharyngeal problem was not yet managed. The most important achievement for the client is to reactivate the speech motor system and re-experience the motor output and somatoafference input associated with speech production. Speaking rate should be kept quite slow initially to allow as much movement-related afference as possible to be realized. Once the basic speech motor patterns have been restored, speaking rate can be adjusted to yield the maximum intelligibility for the client.

Facilitating development of the speech motor system—Methods to facilitate development of the speech motor system in a child with dysarthria would include the above adult considerations *plus* at least the following.

1. Speech motor practice should be with words that are developmentally appropriate. We see unintelligible six-year-olds who appear to have the musculoskeletal and nervous system of three-year-olds. The phonetic material should be geared to their developmental age.

2. Young children are still establishing the motor-afferent linkages (associations, "schemata") to be used as "central programs." Care should be taken in presenting phonetic stimulus materials to maximize early success as these children are forming perhaps the single most important mechanism of the speech motor system, viz., the internal associations of what it feels like to make the movements that generate the acoustics just produced.

3. In the absence of data to the contrary, it seems advantageous to use words as stimuli whenever possible. "One of the predictions from the schema theory is that the subject who receives variable practice develops a strong schema for motor production enabling him to more effectively generate *novel movements*. Now, since the schema refers to a *complex set of relations*, it would seem, for example, that in devising any training programme for schema development, it would make sense to know which of these relationships are weak, i.e., what are the *dimensions of control* which the subject currently cannot handle" (Whiting, 1980, p. 548; italics mine). The most direct evidence we have of poorly controlled dimensions would seem to be the abnormalities in the speech movements. Elicitation

of more correct movements with carefully selected word stimuli would seem most appropriate for facilitating the "set of relationships" between thoughts, words, movements, acoustics, and somatoafference.

4. A final consideration for children relates to the importance of speech in the development of "higher mental functions." It would seem important that language and other cognitive therapies be coupled with speech motor practice. Whereas the practice of the best possible speech is important, its practice in a "thoughtful" environment should be even more helpful in establishing the 'thought to speech' transformations that have formed a central theme in this presentation.

SUMMARY

Data from the past ten to fifteen years on the control of speech production and other motor systems reveal a fast, adaptive nervous system that appears capable of almost instantaneous construction of novel motor acts to express human thoughts through action. The precise neural mechanisms that are used to generate speech motor acts remain unknown for the most part. It is important clinically to be aware of alternative hypotheses about the neural basis of speech motor control when considering (1) what you ask the client to do during the speech examination, (2) how you interpret her or his behavior, and (3) the resultant decisions to be made regarding treatment.

NOTES

[1] "Adaptive control is loosely defined as any control that changes to meet changing needs . . . Thus, a well-designed adaptive system should continue to improve its performance based on past experience and readily adjust to new situations. For this reason, adaptive control is equated with learning" (Houk and Zev Rymer, 1981, p. 261).

[2] This concept is highly similar to that of "functional systems" (see Anokhin, 1974).

[3] Neocortical structures are not confined to cerebral cortex. They include at least the newer portions of the striatum, thalamus, and cerebellum (see review in Netsell, 1982).

[4] For discussions of "schema" in speech motor control, see Kent (1981) and Kent and Minifie (1977).

REFERENCES

Abbs, J., & Cole, K. Consideration of bulbar and suprabulbar efferent influences upon speech motor coordination. In S. Grillner, B. Lindblom, J. Lubker, & A. Persson (Eds.), *Speech motor control.* Elmsford, NY: Pergamon Press, 1982.

Anokhin, P. *Biology and neurophysiology of the conditioned reflex and its role in adaptive behavior.* Elmsford, NY: Pergamon Press, 1974.

Bernstein, N. *Coordination and regulation of movements.* Elmsford, NY: Pergamon Press, 1967.

Brooks, V. *Handbook of physiology: The nervous system, vol. 11, motor control.* Bethesda, MD: American Psychological Society, 1981.

Brown, J. Language representation in the brain. In H.D. Steklis & M.J. Raleigh (Eds.), *Neurogiology of social communication in primates: An evolutionary perspective.* New York: Academic Press, 1979.

Burke, R. Motor units. Anatomy, physiology, and functional organization. In V. Brooks (Ed.), *Handbook of physiology: The nervous system, vol. 11, motor control.* Bethesda, MD: American Physiological Society, 1981.

Capute, A., Shapiro, B., Palmer, F., Accardo, P., & Wachtel, R. Primitive reflexes: A factor in nonverval language in early infancy, In R. Stark (Ed.), *Language behavior in infancy and early childhood.* New York: Elsevier/North Holland, 1981.

Cole, K. *An empirical re-evaluation of minimum voluntary afferent-to-efferent pathway latencies in the orofacial system.* Unpublished master's thesis, University of Wisconsin, 1981.

Dubner, R., Sessle, B., & Storey, A. Peripheral components of motor control. In R. Dubner, B. Sessle, & A. Storey (Eds.), *The neural basis of oral and facial function.* New York: Plenum Press, 1978.

Fry, D. The control of speech and voice. In H. Kalmus (Ed.) *Regulation and control in living systems.* New York: John Wiley & Sons, 1966.

Grillner, S. Possible analogies in the control of innate motor acts and the production of sound in speech. In S. Grillner, B. Lindblom, J. Lubker, & A. Persson (Eds.). *Speech motor control.* Elmsford, NY: Pergamon Press, 1982.

Gurfinkel, V., & Yu S. Levik. Sensory complexes and sensorimotor organization. *Fiziologiya Cheloveka,* 1979, *5,* 399-414.

Hardy, J. Suggestions for physiological research in dysarthria. *Cortex,* 1967, *3,* 128-156.

Hardy, J. Development of neuromuscular systems underlying speech production. In *Speech and the dentofacial complex: The state of the art, ASHA Reports,* 1970, *5,* 49-68.

Hessler, R. The thalmic regulation of muscle tone and the speech of movements. In D. Perpera & M. Yahr (Eds.), *The thalamus.* New York: Columbia University Press, 1966.

Hixon, T. Speech breathing kinematics and mechanism inferences therefrom. In S. Grillner, B. Lindblom, J. Lubker, & A. Persson (Eds.), *Speech motor control.* Elmsford, NY: Pergamon Press, 1982.

Houk, J., & Rymer, W. Neural control of muscle length and tension. In V. Brooks (Ed.), *Handbook of physiology: The nervous system, vol. 11, motor control.* Bethesda, MD: American Physiological Society, 1981.

Kelso, J. Contrasting perspectives on order and regulation in movement. In A. Baddeley & J. Long (Eds.), *Attention and performance IX.* Hillsdale, NJ: Lawrence Erlbaum, 1981.

Kent, R. Sensorimotor aspects of speech development. In R. Aslin, J. Alberts, & M. Petersen (Eds.), *Development of perception: Psychobiological perspectives* (Vol. 1). New York: Academic Press, 1981.

Kent, R., & Minifie, F. Coarticulation in recent speech production models. *Journal of Phonetics,* 1977, *5,* 115-133.

Kent, R., & Moll, K. Articulatory timing in selected consonant sequences. *Brain and Language,* 1975, *2,* 304-323.

Ladefoged, P., DeClerk, J., Lindau, M., & Papcun, G. An auditory-motor theory of speech production, *UCLA working papers in phonetics*, 1972, *22*, 48-75.

Luria, A. *Higher cortical function in man*. New York: Basic Books, 1980.

Luschei, E., & Goldberg, L. Neural mechanisms of mandibular control: Mastication and voluntary biting. In V. Brooks (Ed.), *Handbook of physiology: The nervous system, vol. 11, motor control*. Bethesda, MD: American Physiological Society, 1981.

MacLean, P. The triune brain, emotion and scientific bias. In F.O. Schmitt (Ed.), *The neurosciences: Second study program*. New York: Rockefeller University Press, 1970.

MacNeilage, P. Motor control of serial ordering of speech. *Psychological Review*, 1970, *77*, 181-196.

Mateer, K. Asymmetric effects of thalamic stimulation on rate of speech. *Neuropsychologica*, 1978, *16*, 497-499.

Miller, J., & Hardy, J. Considerations in evaluating dysarthria. Paper presented at the meeting of the American Speech and Hearing Association, New York, 1962.

Mountcastle, V. An organizing principle for cerebral function: The unit module and the distributed system. In G. Edleman & V. Mountcastle (Eds.), *The mindful brain*. Cambridge: MIT Press, 1978.

Mysak E. *Pathologies of speech systems*. Baltimore: Williams and Wilkens Co., 1976.

Mysak, E. *Neurospeech therapy for the cerebral palsied: A neuroevolutional approach*. New York: Teachers College Press, 1980.

Netsell, R. Physiological bases of dysarthria. Final report, Research Grant NS 09627, National Institutes of Health. Bethesda, MD, 1976.

Netsell, R. Speech motor control: Searching for specialized neural mechanisms. Paper presented to the Meeting on Speech motor control, Madison, WI: 1980.

Netsell, R. Speech motor control and selected neurologic disorders. In S. Grillner, B. Lindblom, J. Lubker, & A. Persson (Eds.), *Speech Motor Control.* Elmsford, NY: Pergamon Press, 1982.

Netsell, R., Kent, R., & Abbs, J. The organization and reorganization of speech movements. Paper presented at the meeting of the Society for Neurosciences, Cincinnati: 1980.

Ojemann, G., & Mateer, C. Cortical and subcortical organization of human communication: Evidence from stimulation studies. In H.D. Steklis & M.J. Raleigh (Eds.), *Communication in primates: An evolutionary perspective.* New York: Academic Press, 1979.

Ojemann, G., & Ward, A. Speech representation in ventrolateral thalamus. *Brain,* 1980, *94,* 669-680.

Rack, P. Limitations of somatosensory feedback in control of posture and movements. In V. Brooks (Ed.), *Handbook of physiology: The nervous system, vol. 11, motor control.* Bethesda, MD: American Physiological Society, 1981.

Rosenbek, J., & LaPointe, L. The dysarthrias: Description, diagnosis and treatment. In D. Johns (Ed.), *Clinical management of neurogenic communication disorders.* Boston: Little, Brown and Co., 1978.

Shaughnessy, A., Lotz, W., & Netsell, R. Laryngeal resistence for syllable series and word productions. Paper presented at the meeting of the American Speech-Language-Hearing Association, Los Angeles, 1981.

Smitheran, J., & Hixon, T. A clinical method for estimating laryngeal airway resistance during vowel productions. *Journal of Speech and Hearing Disorders,* 1981, *46,* 138-146.

Whiting, H. Dimensions of control in motor learning. In G. Stelmach & J. Requin (Eds.), *Tutorials in motor behavior.* New York: North-Holland Publishing Co., 1980.

Wolff, P. Theoretical issues in the development of motor skills. Symposium on Development Disabilities in the Pre-School Child, Johnson & Johnson Baby Products, Chicago, 1979.

ACKNOWLEDGEMENTS

Raymond Kent provided helpful comments on an earlier version of this paper. This work was supported by the Boys Town Institute for Communication Disorders in Children and the National Institutes of Health.

2

Differential Speech Motor Subsystem Impairments with Suprabulbar Lesions: Neurophysiological Framework and Supporting Data

James H. Abbs
Chauncey J. Hunker
Steven M. Barlow

INTRODUCTION AND RATIONALE

Recent developments in the treatment of dysarthria have involved increased emphasis upon focused physical intervention, including biofeedback, palatal lifts, posturing, abdominal binding, etc. (see Hixon, 1975; Netsell and Daniel, 1979; Rubow and Netsell, 1979; Rubow, 1981). These physically oriented treatments demand detailed assessment information concerning the speech mechanism pathophysiology in each patient (Netsell, 1979). For example, it is difficult to justify general relaxation biofeedback to reduce muscle tone if the nature, degree and distribution of that increased tone is not specified empirically. Indeed, the success of many such intervention techniques may rely as much on detailed knowledge of the motor pathophysiology as on the techniques themselves. Unfortunately, the degree of insight provided by current clinical assessment procedures concerning the actual physiological impairment has not been evaluated systematically.

As illustrated in Figure 2-1, state-of-the-art assessment procedures as they are used routinely in most clinical settings, appear to involve several serial steps in determining the apparent pathophysiology. These are: (1) auditory-perceptual evaluation of the dysarthric speech patterns with attempts, via speech task manipulations, to determine the relative degree of impairment in the major components of the speech production system (i.e., respiratory, phonatory, articulatory), (2) ["differential diagnosis" identification of the apparent syndrome(s), using formal or informal auditory-perceptual categorization procedures (e.g., Darley, Aronson, and Brown, 1969a, b, 1975), and (3) inferences as to the movement and muscle contraction impairment manifestations in the speech production system, based on (a) concurrent neurological evaluations of the limb motor system and or (b) classical, stereotypic descriptions of the syndrome-associated limb ʼpathophysiology as outlined in neurological literature. For example, if the differential diagnosis yields the identification of hypokinetic dysarthria (Parkinson's disease), it is inferred (or assumed) that the speech motor impairment is a manifestation of rigidity, hypo/bradykinesia and/or resting tremor in the muscles and movements of the speech production system. This pathophysiological profile is, of course, the classical one offered in traditional neurological texts for the limbs (Patton, Sudsten, Crill, and Swanson, 1976).[1] Hence, this assessment process, if we have characterized it appropriately, is based upon two fundamental and related assumptions. The first of these is that limb pathophysiology provides a valid basis for making inferences to associated speech motor problems. That is, there appears to be an implicit assumption that the pathophysiology of a movement disorder in its stereotypic form is manifest across limb and speech motor subsystems. This, of course, highlights the second assumption, namely, that the motor subsystems of the speech production system likewise are impaired uniformly as a result of particular suprabulbar/supraspinal injury, i.e., the lips, tongue, jaw, larynx, etc., will show similar patterns of pathophysiology.

Our interest in these issues was stimulated by the multi-component representation of the speech production system that Netsell (1971) proposed as a guiding framework for physiological assessment and treatment of motor speech disorders. Our version of this representation with a schematic inclusion of the underlying nervous system is illustrated in Figure 2-2.

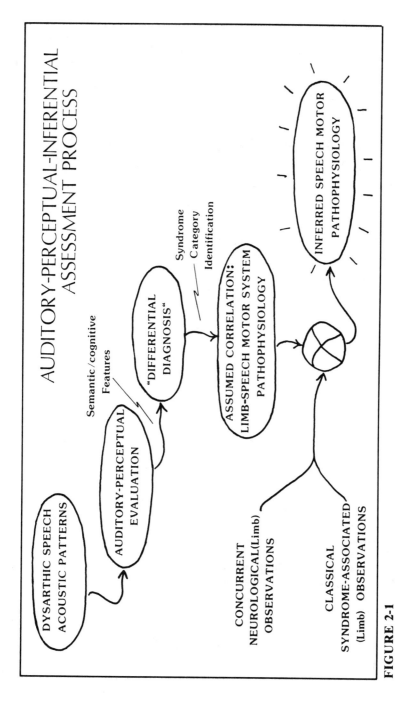

FIGURE 2-1
A schematic illustration of the auditory perceptual-inferential assessment procedure for determining speech motor pathophysiology in dysarthria

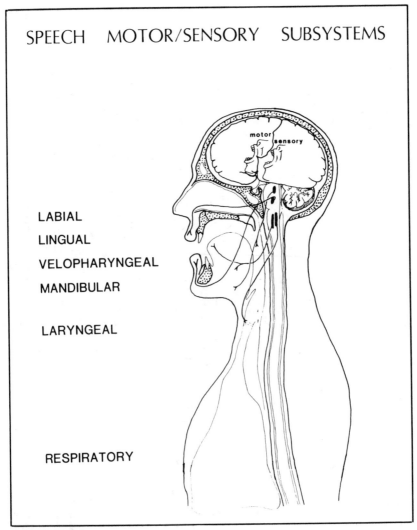

SPEECH   MOTOR/SENSORY   SUBSYSTEMS

LABIAL

LINGUAL

VELOPHARYNGEAL

MANDIBULAR

LARYNGEAL

RESPIRATORY

FIGURE 2-2
A schematic representation of the multiple motor subsystems of the speech production system re: assessment of dysarthria

As noted, this multi-component orientation is based upon the argument that assessment of different speech motor subsystems is necessary to develop an optimal program of component-focused rehabilitation. This approach makes a great deal of sense in evaluating potential lower motoneuron disorders where one might anticipate differential subsystem impairments due to damage in some cranial nerves and not others. At issue, however, is whether or not it is similarly useful to conduct such multiple subsystem assessment in dysarthrias of suprabulbar origin. If suprabulbar lesions uniformly influence all the motor subsystems of the speech production system in the same manner, it may be unnecessary to evaluate more than one speech motor subsystem. For example, one could observe the control impairments in the most accessible speech motor subsystems—e.g., the lips—and make inferences as to the control impairments in the jaw, tongue, larynx, velum, etc. However, if this assumption is incorrect, that is, if a suprabulbar lesion results in non-uniform control impairments across the speech motor subsystems, inferences regarding the speech motor control profile cannot be made from observations of a single motor subcomponent. Obviously, it also would be difficult to make parallel inferences from limb motor impairments, as classically defined, to presumed impairments in the orofacial system, (see Darley, Aronson, and Brown, 1975). The key issue, in determining the general validity of either the multiple speech component or the auditory-perceptual-inferential assessment approaches, is whether the suprabulbar structures play the same controlling role for all of the speech motor subsystems. In short, *is the movement control required by the CNS uniform in nature for the limbs, abdomen, rib cage, larynx, pharynx, jaw, tongue, lips, etc.?* If the answer to this question is negative and the control requirements are substantial, then damage at suprabulbar levels should yield non-uniform impairments among cranial and spinal motor subsystems. There are several ways to approach these issues, the major avenues being analytic and empirical. In the present paper, we would like to share the outcome of our analytic considerations—i.e., examination of underlying limb and speech production subsystem motor physiology—and augment this theoretical evaluation with some empirical physiological observations of speech motor subsystem dysfunctions in subjects with "pure" suprabulbar impairments.

MOTOR CONTROL IMPLICATIONS OF
SUBSYSTEM CHARACTERISTICS

Analytically, it is useful to take a *systems physiology* approach in determining the potential role of the central nervous system in controlling the different speech and spinal motor subsystems (see Milhorn, 1966; Talbot and Gessner, 1973; Partridge, 1976; Robinson, 1981). The systems approach is particularly well-suited to this analysis because it requires that

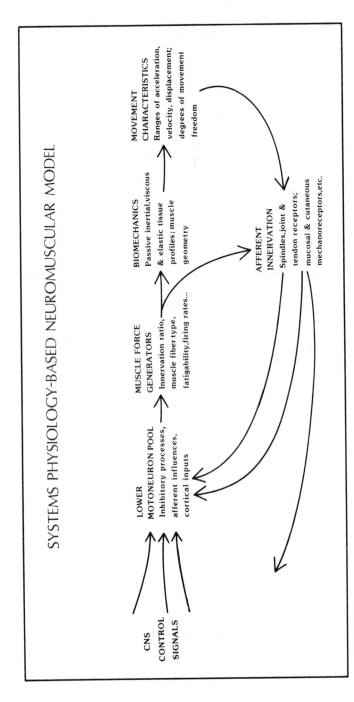

FIGURE 2-3
A flow diagram representation of the major features of a systems physiology model of a neuromuscular system

the major functional subsystem properties be identified and evaluated. In short, this analysis asks what critical motor subsystem characteristics must be considered for central nervous system control? (Muller, Abbs, and Kennedy, 1981). If these critical characteristics are the same for different motor subsystems, we have reason to argue for control uniformity. The major components of a stereotypic systems physiology-based neuromuscular model are represented in Figure 2-3.

As shown, these include: (1) system movement characteristics, e.g., acceleration, velocity, and range of movement, etc.: (2) system biomechanics, multi-muscle geometry, muscle force generation characteristics, passive mechanics including inertial, elastic, and viscous properties, (3) efferent innervation of the muscles, e.g., innervation ratio, fiber histochemical properties, etc., (4) sensory innveration—the density and presence of muscle spindles, tendon organs, joint receptors, and cutaneous mucosal mechanoreceptors—and (5) the pattern of efferent and afferent influences impinging upon the lower motoneuron pool, including the distribution and nature of peripheral afferent influences, reciprocal recurrent inhibition processes and inputs from descending cortical pathways. These system physiology properties have been shown to be of major significance in discerning how particular motor systems are controlled by suprabulbar/supraspinal mechanisms. This is reflected in a substantial body of empirical evidence from experimental and mathematical analyses of motor systems in animals and man (see Houk, 1972; Neilson, Andrews, Guitar, and Quinn, 1979; Robinson, 1981; Houk and Rymer, 1981; Stein, 1982).

In applying this analysis framework to speech and limb motor subsystems, it is apparent that there are a number of very significant physiological and neurophysiological differences. To illustrate the basis for this argument, it is useful to consider the neuromuscular system profiles for some speech and upper limb motor subsystems. In the context of the framework presented in Figure 2-3, we will first examine the major movement and biomechanical characteristics of these subsystems. The biomechanical properties of motor systems are extremely important in dictating the muscle contraction patterns (and hence CNS control signals) required to produce certain patterns of movement (cf. Abbs and Eilenberg, 1976). For example, mass (inertial) properties have a direct and undeniable Newtonian influence upon the force required to get a movement up to a certain velocity (i.e., acceleration). Likewise, the "fluid friction" (viscosity) found in all or most biological tissues demands proportional increases in muscle force as greater movement velocities are required. Hence, while slow movements of two motor subsystems can be driven in a comparable manner (re: the muscle contraction-CNS control signal patterns), increases in acceleration and/or velocity may require very different control signals depending upon the relative magnitudes of inherent inertia and viscosity (Abbs and Muller, 1980). In relation to biomechanical comparisons of the lips, tongue, upper limbs, etc., we know that the lips do not have a significant inertial (mass) component while these other movement systems require inclusion of intertia in their biomechanical profile (Abbs and Muller, 1980). It may be significant that the movements of the lips are generally more rapid than those of these other structures.

Additional biomechanical differences between these systems are related to the presence and nature of connective tissue restraints. That is, the jaw and upper limbs have tendons, ligaments, and move through trajectories circumscribed by joints. By contrast, the lip musculature is without joint constraints and does not have tendonous or ligamentous connective tissue; moreover, the facial muscles are not separated by facial sheaths. Like the lips, the tongue intrinsic muscle structure is without typical connective tissue and the outer covering of this articulator plays a different connective role than individual muscle tendons and facial sheaths. The potential influence of these movements and biomechanical characteristics upon control requirements is apparent when one considers work on the control of eye movements where different central nervous system mechanisms have been implicated for rapid movements (saccadic), slow movements (smooth pursuit), and static positioning (fixation). That is, within the occular system, there are documented neuroanatomical differences in the control network that vary as a function of movement demands (Robinson, 1981). Movement-dependent neural control differences also have been suggested by Kornhuber (1975) who proposed that slow, postural movements are highly dependent on the basal ganglia while fast, "ballistic" movements are more dependent upon the cerebellar circuits. Obviously, if Kornhuber's notion is correct, basal ganglia (or cerebellar) lesions should cause very different impairments among the various speech or limb motor or limb motor subsystems, depending upon whether their movements are slow or fast.

Applying this analysis to sensory innervation in these motor subsystems (re: Figure 2-3), it is of note that while the jaw and upper limbs have muscle spindles, joint, and tendon receptors (Harrison and Corbin, 1942; Kubota, Masegi, and Osani, 1974; Lund, Richmond, Touloumis, Patry, and Lemarre, 1978); the lips have none of these (Lovell, Sutton, and Lindeman, 1977; Folkins and Larson, 1978; and the tongue has only muscle spindles (Cooper, 1953; Bowman and Combs, 1968; Fitzgerald and Sachithanandan, 1979). The larynx apparently has each of these receptors (Lucas Keene, 1961; Baken, 1971; Larson, Sutton and Lindeman, 1974), as in the case of the jaw. A major difference between the jaw and upper limbs is that while the jaw closing muscles are densely supplied with muscle spindles, very few, if any, appear to be present in the jaw opening muscles (Lund, Richmond, Touloumis, Patry, and Lamarre, 1978); viz., it doesn't appear that there is a comparable spindle density difference between antagonistic muscles in the upper limbs. Clearly, if we posit a role of any or all of these afferent systems in the control of movement, their absence in a particular motor subsystem requires a parallel difference in the required CNS control signals (see Houk and Rymer, 1981; Muller, Abbs and Kennedy, 1981).

Another important factor, also noted in Figure 2-3, is the nature of the influences impinging upon the lower motoneuron pool; by definition these influences must determine the final pattern of efferent signals to the muscle. With regard to afferent influences on the lower motoneurons, it is notable that while spindles in the jaw and upper limbs make monosynaptic connections, spindle afferents from the larynx and tongue are not so configured (Bowman and Combs, 1968; Bratzlavsky and vander Eecken, 1974; Neilson, Andrews, Guitar, and Quinn, 1979). Labial and lingual cutaneous and mucosal mechanoreceptor influences on motoneurons are known to be polysynaptic. However, it appears doubtful that lingual muscle spindles have any direct autogenic influence on the lingual motoneurons. Further, while spindle primary (Ia) afferents in the limbs make connections to all motoneurons in a muscle, in the jaw spindles appear to make connections only to small motoneurons (Appenteng, O'Donovan, Somjen, Stephens, and Taylor, 1978). The nervous system control implications of these variable afferent influences upon the lower motoneuron pool appear particularly significant, especially with regard to such phenomena as the size principle of motoneuron recruitment (see Henneman, Somjen, and Carpenter, 1965a, b; Henneman, 1975; Burke, 1981); for example, the differential influences of spindle feedback on jaw motoneurons may influence recruitment order. Inasmuch as the lips do not have spindles influencing the lower motoneuron pool, these muscles also are likely to show differences in motoneuron recruitment patterns in comparison to the limbs and jaw. While patterns of recurrent and reciprocal inhibition are manifest for the upper limbs via lower motoneuron interactions with collaterals to inhibitory interneurons and spindle afferents, parallel processes do not appear to be operating for the cranial nerves; rather, it appears that control of these important inhibitory patterns is regulated more centrally (Penders and Delwaide, 1973; Shahani and Young, 1973; Dubner, Sessle, and Storey, 1978). Of major importance may be the potentially related fact that in primates (including man) motoneurons of the lips, jaw, and tongue muscles receive monosynaptic inputs from corticomotor sites, (Watson, 1973; Kuypers, 1958) while the motoneurons of the larynx, respiratory system, and upper limbs (independent of the digits) do not (Carpenter, 1976).

These neurophysiological and neuroanatomical differences are almost irrefutable evidence that the CNS does not control the spinal and cranial systems nor their respective motor subsystems in the same manner. Indeed a differential neuromuscular substrate appears to be the rule rather than the exception; the motorsensory and sensorimotor homunculi make this conclusion painfully obvious. The inescapable prediction is that if there is damage to a certain part of the central nervous system at a suprabulbar/supraspinal level, the result will be impairments in movement and muscle contraction that are different among the speech production subsystems and the limbs. For example, hypo- and hyper-gamma motor drive to muscle spindles, loss or aberrations in recurrent inhibition, and impairment of selective influences on motoneuron pool recruitment patterns have all enjoyed some popularity as partial pathogenic explanations for spasticity, rigidity, tremor, ataxia, hypotonia, dysmetria, and asthenia. If some of these explanations are even partially correct, and the implicated physiological processes (e.g., presence of spindles, operation of recurrent inhibition) differ from one motor subsystem to another, then the motor pathophysiology must differ as well. While this hypothesis has some support in observations of differential muscle contraction impairments between the upper and lower limbs, e.g., degrees of spasticity, rigidity, tremor, etc., there is a paucity of compatable physiological data that address the possibility of such differential impairment profiles among the motor subsystems of the speech production mechanism.

Based on this theoretical rationale and the importance for treatment noted previously, we have focused in the last three to four years on obtaining speech motor subsystem impairment profiles in subjects with Parkinson's disease, congenital spasticity, and cerebellar damage. While the scope of this paper does not permit presentation of all the findings obtained to date, a review of our major results suffices to address the issue of motor subsystem impairment differences with these particular populations. These data thus represent the empirical analysis component of this paper, alluded to previously.

PATHOPHYSIOLOGICAL PROFILES
OF THE SPEECH MOTOR SUBSYSTEMS

A major methodological consideration in evaluating the validity of differential subsystem impairments is assurance that the dysarthric subjects studied present "pure" and uncontaminated signs of their representative syndrome category. We have taken a number of special precautions in this regard, including (1) two independent neurological evaluations, i.e., one by a clinical neurologist and a second one by a laboratory staff research neurologist, (2) complete oral-peripheral speech and non-speech evaluation by a research speech pathologist, and (3) elimination of any subjects showing even mild signs of a "mixed" neurological disease. We were particularly careful to eliminate any subjects with secondary bulbar/lower motoneuron signs as manifest by standard clinical evaluations. In short, we are confident that the subjects described in the discussions that follow presented stereotypic neurological profiles in limb and orofacial pathophysiology.

Parkinsonian Dysarthria

In Parkinson patients, the major signs of the motor impairment are said to include muscle rigidity and hypokinesia, the latter characterized by a reduction in the range of movement. In a series of experiments (Hunker, Abbs, and Barlow, 1982), we quantitatively examined the relationship between these two components of the movement disorder in the labial muscles of Parkinson and normal subjects. The four Parkinson subjects were ranked according to the severity of their dysarthria, which ranged from moderately severe to mild (respectively labeled subjects, P1, P2, P3, and P4). Labial muscle rigidity was quantified by applying known forces (ΔF) and observing the resultant displacement (ΔX), using the transduction system illustrated in Figure 2-4.

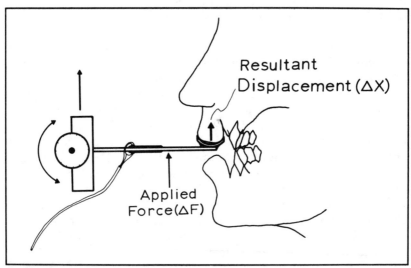

FIGURE 2-4
A schematic illustration of the strain gauge force transducer mounted on a
rack and pinion
* The orientation of the cantilever beam could be configured to displace the upper lip or lower lip a discrete
vertical distance, and the force required to produce the displacement simultaneously measured.

By plotting these measures, as shown in Figure 2-5 A,B for the upper and
lower lips, it was observed that the displacements increased linearly with
the applied forces. The slopes of these curves provided a quantitative index
of labial muscle stiffness ($\Delta F / \Delta X$) and yielded the stiffness coefficients.
Because the data from the normal subjects were remarkably similar, the
values from these subjects were pooled and fitted to a single curve.

As is apparent in Figure 2-5A, lower lip stiffness of all Parkinson subjects
was significantly greater than the normal subjects. As shown in Figure 2-
5B, Parkinson dysarthrics P1 and P2 (the two most severe subjects)
showed abnormal stiffness in the upper lip; by contrast, P3 and P4 had
normal values, viz., abnormal stiffness (rigidity) was manifested
differentially between the upper and lower lips in these latter subjects.

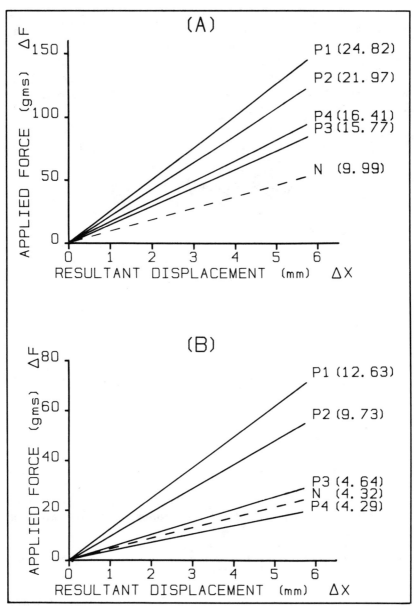

FIGURE 2-5
Lip stiffness curves and the respective stiffness coefficients for all subjects
*(A) shows those of the lower lip and (B) those of the upper lip.

In parallel, labial speech movements were observed in these same Parkinson subjects to evaluate hypokinesia. Bilabial displacement magnitudes were obtained by measuring the excursion of the upper and lower lips for the vowel to consonant movements in "Bobby" and "poppy" (distance between points A and B in Figure 2-6) as recorded by a headmounted lip and jaw movement transduction system (Barlow, Cole, Abbs, in press).

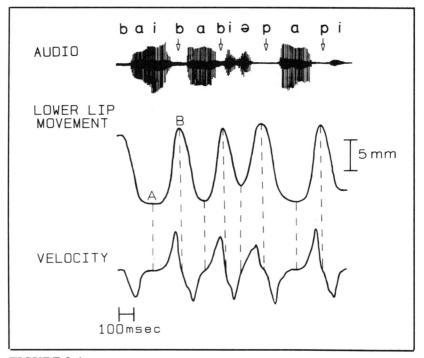

FIGURE 2-6
Oscillographic recordings of speech audio, lower lip movement and velocity for the production of "Buy Bobby a poppy" (bai b a bi ə p a pi) by a normal speaker.*

*Points of measurement of the bilabial stops in "babi" and "papi": A maximum lip opening corresponding to zero velocity, and B-maximum lip closure corresponding to zero velocity. The distance between these maximum amplitudes was measured as an index of lip displacement magnitude.

Figure 2-7 shows the results of these measurements for the upper and lower lips. For subjects P1 and P2, the range of both upper and lower lip movement was significantly less than normal. However, in parallel with the stiffness observations in subjects P3 and P4, the displacements of the upper lip were normal, while those of the lower lip were reduced.

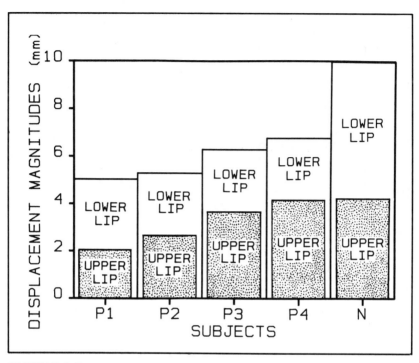

FIGURE 2-7
A graphic comparison of upper and lower lip displacement magnitudes for the bilabial stops for all subjects

By combining the results of these two experiments, it was obvious that labial rigidity was consistently correlated with decrements in the range of lip movement. Figure 2-8A, B show plots of the stiffness coefficients for all subjects as a function of mean displacement magnitudes for the lower and upper lip, respectively.

These plots offer a qualitative indication that increased muscle tone is accompanied by decrements in the range of lip movement and that in the Parkinson subjects there is both differential stiffness and a differential reduction in the range of lip movement.

Several additional conclusions are forced by these data. The first is that, while muscle rigidity and hypokinesia are parameters of the pathophysiology of the limb musculature in Parkinson patients, one can not assume that they are present uniformly in the speech motor subsystems without specific speech-nonspeech observations. Second, these observations point up the limitations of perceptual and acoustical analysis.

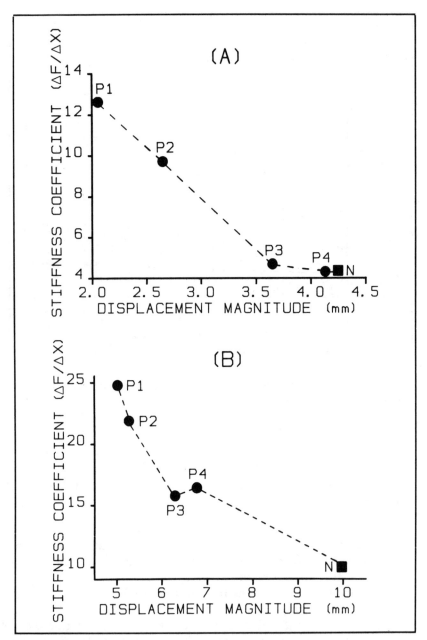

FIGURE 2-8A, B
The relationship between the stiffness coefficients and the mean displacement magnitudes for the upper lip (A) and lower lip (B) for all subjects

That is, if one were to perceptually or acoustically note frication of bilabial stop consonants, as is frequently observed in Parkinsonian dysarthria (see Canter, 1963; Logemann, Fisher, Boshes, and Blonsky, 1978; Kent and Netsell, 1979; Logemann and Fisher, 1981), it would be impossible to determine whether the misarticulations were due to: (1) reduced range of lower lip movement, (2) reduced range of both upper and lower lip movements, (3) reduced range of upper lip, lower lip, and jaw movements, and/or (4) errors in timing and discoordination between the upper lip, lower lip and jaw, as might be expected with differential impairments in bilabial movement. Finally, these observations indicate the utility of the non-speech measures of the speech production system to predict speech impairments; as such, these results directly contradict suggestions and interpretations regarding the assessment value of non-speech measures by Hixon and Hardy (1964) and Hardy (1970).

Another set of data obtained with Parkinson subjects concerned the control of fine muscle contraction forces in the lips, tongue and jaw using the set of three force transducers shown in Figure 2-9 (Barlow and Abbs, in press).

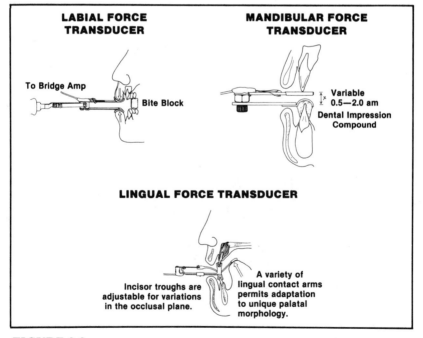

FIGURE 2-9
Line illustration of labial, lingual, and mandibular force transducers
*after Barlow and Abbs, in press.

For these measures, the subjects are asked to produce prespecified levels of steady force, with visual feedback from a storage oscilloscope. These levels were chosen to approximate the forces necessary for speech movements; we were not concerned with maximum force, per se. Figure 2-10 is a set of tongue elevation force traces obtained from a normal subject and a Parkinson dysarthric.

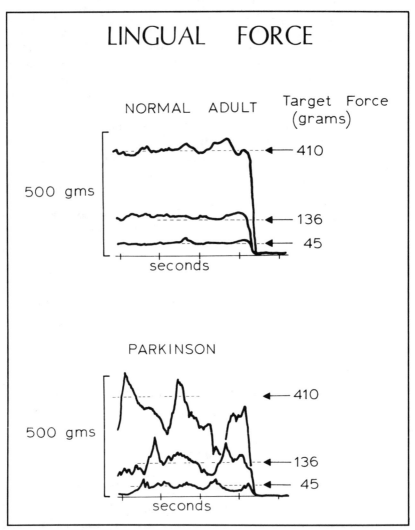

FIGURE 2-10
Lingual contraction forces from a normal and a Parkinson dysarthric

For the normal subject, the stability of force generation was only minimally influenced by increasing the force level. In contrast, the Parkinson subject showed substantially more instability in producing steady tongue elevation forces at each end of the targeted performance levels. If all subsystems were similarly impaired in this Parkinson subject, one would expect to see a parallel of instability for the lips and jaw. Figure 2-11 contrasts sustained low level forces generated by the lips, jaw, and tongue from these same two subjects.

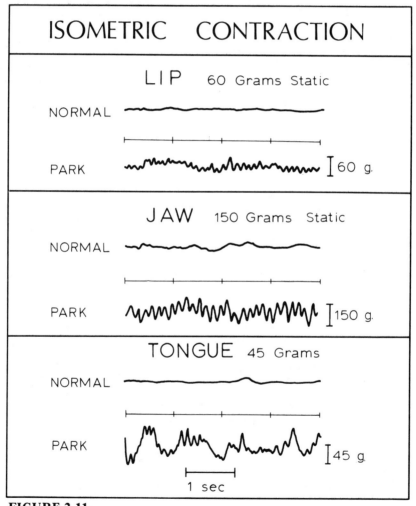

FIGURE 2-11
Labial, mandibular, and lingual contraction forces from a normal and Parkinson dysarthric

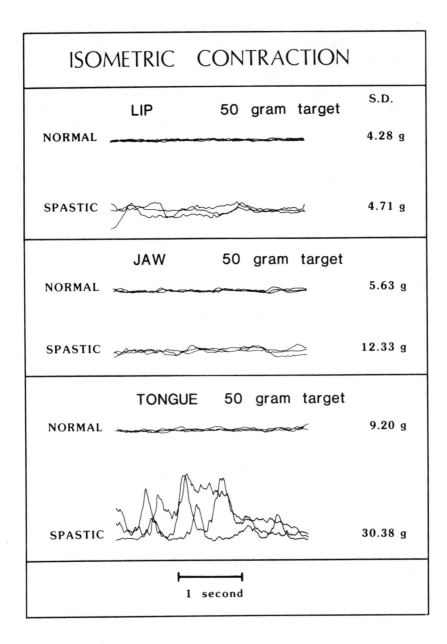

FIGURE 2-12
Labial, mandibular, and lingual contraction forces from a normal subject
and a spastic cerebral-palsied adult subject

While the tongue forces in the Parkinson subject are characterized primarily by large fluctuations and general instability, as before, the lips and jaw were generally stable with tremor being the major abnormal/normal distinction. Also apparent in Figure 2-11 are differences in tremor between the lips and jaw. In this particular subject, the lip has a tremor frequency ranging from 8-9 Hz, while the jaw has a lower tremor frequency (6 Hz). These subsystem differences in the generation of muscle contraction forces and in their tremor frequencies further indicate the significant impairment variation across these articulatory subsystems. These data speak, as well, to the potential limitations in perceptual, acoustical and/or aerodynamic assessment. For example, if lingual consonants are lacking in precision, as often is suggested in the Parkinson population, it would appear very difficult to ascertain, using perceptual, acoustic and/or aerodynamic measures, whether the imprecision was due to lingual or mandibular control impairments. The implication is strong that these more global observations of speech production may not provide enough information to identify impairments which are differentially distributed across the speech motor subsystems.

Congenital Spasticity and Dysarthria

Parallel observations of fine muscle force control have been made in spastic cerebral palsy adults. Figure 2-12 contrasts force control patterns obtained from the lips, jaw and tongue.

With this subject, the greatest control instability was observed in the tongue, a pattern similar to that of the Parkinson subject discussed previously. By contrast, lip and jaw control for this subject are relatively impaired. Figure 2-13 shows another articulatory force control impairment pattern seen in this population.

As is apparent in this subject, the lips and tongue show the greatest instability at high force levels (in force ranges that are not particularly important for the small, fine contractions for speech), while jaw instability is greatest at very low force levels, i.e., the jaw instability is in direct contrast to the lips and tongue. Our observations in this congenital spastic population further demonstrate support for the differential subsystem impairment hypothesis, with evidence for motor control differences in both degree and kind. Also, as with the Parkinson dysarthrics, it is apparent that there is not a stereotypic profile of subsystem impairment, even in populations where neurological examinations and perceptual evaluations

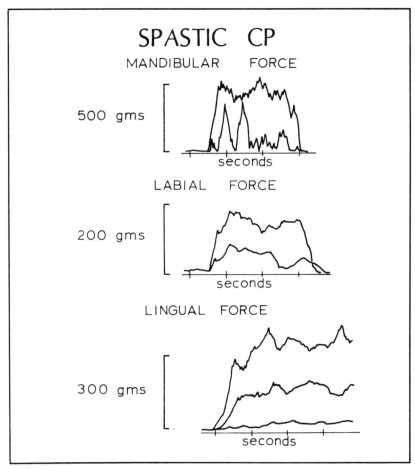

FIGURE 2-13
Mandibular labial, and lingual contraction forces for a spastic cerebral-palsied adult subject

yield the same general diagnosis.

A methodological issue regarding these differential impairment profiles is raised when considering earlier arguments suggesting that observations of non-speech control impairments in this population are not indicative or predictive of speech motor impairments. (see Hixon and Hardy, 1964; Hardy, 1970). In the subject profiled in Figure 2-12, it was decided to informally test this notion by observing patterns of speech with the differentially impaired jaw fixed; a fitted bite-block was placed between the teeth. It was hypothesized that eliminating the jaw instability would improve the overall articulatory control pattern because the jaw might be introducing a disproportionate degree of movement instability into the movement patterns between these closely linked articulators (Barlow and Abbs, 1982). Figure 2-14 shows the result of that procedure.

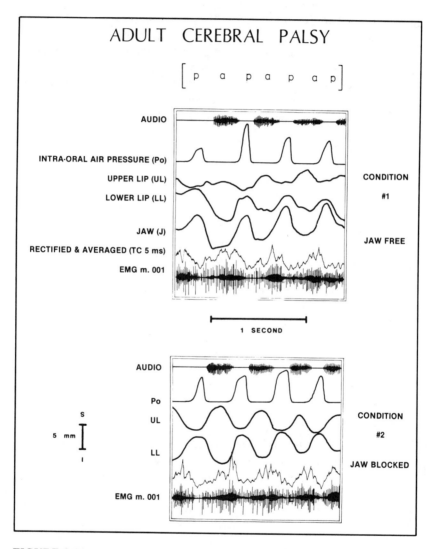

FIGURE 2-14

Physiological signals from a spastic cerebral-palsied adult subject with the jaw free to vary (upper panel) and the jaw fixed (lower panel)

In the upper panel of this figure is an oscillographic record of the speech acoustic signal, intraoral air pressure, upper lip, lower lip, and jaw movement and muscle activity from orbicularis oris for a series of [pa] syllables. The lip and jaw movements are irregular and asymmetric; the inter-coordination pattern is neither consistent nor reciprocal (re: Hughes and Abbs, 1976). Corresponding irregularities are reflected in the magnitudes and duration of the audio signal and intraoral air pressure pulses. The labial muscle EMG is generally undifferentiated, i.e., discrete bursts of muscle activity normally associated with bilabial closure are absent. These patterns are consistent with those previously reported on cerebral-palsied dysarthrics (Kent and Netsell, 1978). The lower panel in Figure 2-14 shows the same set of signals for the bite-block condition. As is apparent, both upper and lower lip movements are more regular with increased excursion and increased velocity, vowels are more uniform in duration (re: the acoustic signal) and the intra-oral air pressures are more consistent in amplitude, duration, and time history. Similarly, the EMG of the orbicularis oris muscle shows a semblance of phasic bursts typically seen in normal productions of bilabial stop gestures of this type.

The observations shown in Figure 2-14 augment the earlier suggestion that perceptual, acoustic, or aerodynamic measures do not provide the information to make inferences to underlying pathophysiology. For example, perceptual, acoustical, or aerodynamic observations of the labial consonant imprecision evidenced in Figure 2-14 would not provide a basis for disambiguating labial vs. mandibular impairment. Also, it is apparent that observations of impairments discernible on non-speech tasks can refine observations made with perceptual, acoustical, or aerodynamic procedures in pointing to the locus of the underlying pathophysiology.

Ataxic Dysarthria

Further empirical evidence supporting differential subsystem impairments within the speech production mechanism has been obtained from subjects with cerebellar involvement. Because of the practical limits of this paper, we will focus upon only one feature of the motor impairments of these subjects, that of "discoordination." Generally, it has been suggested that these subjects display a decomposition of movement in multi-structure movement gesture, like the discoordination of movements around the shoulder, elbow, and wrist associated with pointing (cf. Holmes, 1922). This classical description has led to some individuals who have observed the motor speech disorders associated with this population to suggest that the characteristic dysarthria speech pattern is a

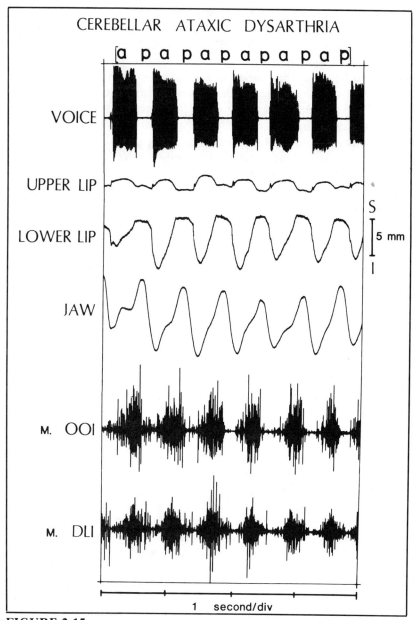

FIGURE 2-15

Upper lip, lower lip, and jaw movement from an ataxic dysarthric subject during production of a series of [pa's]

*EMG from orbicularis oris inferior (OOI) and depressor labii inferior (DLI) was recorded with hooked wire electrodes.

manifestation of a similar pathophysiology; the inference is that the articulators are inappropriately timed and/or overshoot and undershoot intended targets. In the last several years, we have been fortunate enough to find several subjects with pure cerebellar signs in the limbs and associated ataxic dysarthria and, hence, have experimentally examined their speech movements with regard to manifestations of discoordination. Figure 2-15 is a record of voice, upper lip, lower lip, and jaw movement from the same subject studied by Kent and Netsell (1975).

The individual movements are not smoothly executed and are characterized by jerkiness and a general slowness, essentially the classical signs reported by Holmes (1922) and also consistent with the observations of Kent and Netsell (1975). However, despite these aberrations, the upper lip, lower lip, and jaw generally move in phase toward closure (for the bilabial stops) and opening (for associated vowels). If we define coordination as an ability to control the movements of individual sub-components of a complex gesture syngeristically, this particular subject appears to be free from gross discoordination problems between the labial-mandibular subsystems.

In a parallel experiment on the same day, we were able to monitor the performance of the respiratory subsystem in this same subject (Hunker, Bless, and Weismer, 1981). Circumferential size changes of the rib cage and abdomen were independently transduced providing analog signals of chest wall kinematics as well as a calibrated index of total lung volume change during a parallel set of speech and nonspeech tasks. The rib cage and abdominal components of the respiratory subsystem must be coordinated in their respective movements inasmuch as they contribute simultaneously to changes in total lung volume and the production of subglottal air pressures during speech (Hixon, Goldman, and Mead, 1973; Hixon, Mead, and Goldman, 1976). Figure 2-16 shows the rib cage and abdominal displacement patterns for the ataxic dysarthric and a normal speaker, each producing the same sentence twice.

In examining the normal respiratory subsystem pattern, it is apparent that rib cage and abdominal movements are in phase, that is, their respective contributions to lung volume change during the utterance are expiratory and, therefore, complimentary. By contrast, if we examine the pattern of the ataxic speaker, it is apparent that the two normally coordinated components of the respiratory subsystem are moving in opposition or paradoxically. As indicated by opposing arrows (Figure 2-16), on several occasions rib cage contibutions to lung volume change are expiratory at

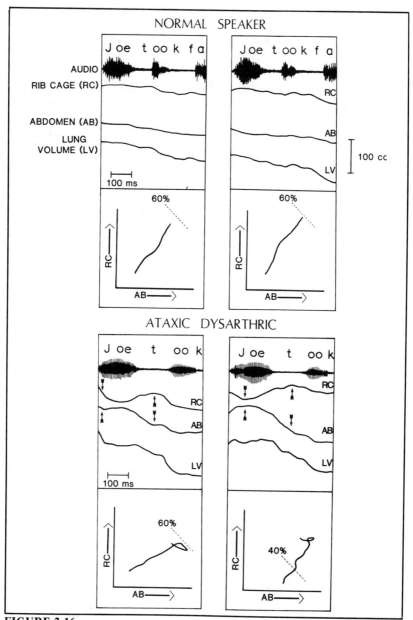

FIGURE 2-16
Abdomen, rib cage, and lung volume changes during the initial portion of the sentence "Joe took father's shoe bench out" for a normal subject and an ataxic dysarthric subject

* Motion-motion diagrams of rib cage and abdominal movements are after Hixon et al., 1973.

the same time abdominal contribution is inspiratory and conversely. As a result of this discoordination between the rib cage and abdomen, there appears to be some interference in lung volume control and perhaps related influences on subglottal pressure. In the case of this ataxic subject, it is apparent that the lip-jaw coordination, as defined previously, is essentially normal. However, coordination of the rib cage and abdomen, in the respiratory subsystem, is aberrant. This example yields a conclusion similar to that of the Parkinson and congenital spastic subjects, namely, that the speech motor subsystems are impaired in a differential manner.

SUMMARY AND CONCLUSIONS

Overall, these physiological observations support the prediction from the systems analysis of orofacial and spinal motor neurophysiology; different speech motor subsystems are controlled differently by the CNS and, hence, suprabulbar lesions yield differential impairments to these subsystems. The implications of these observations in relation to assessments and treatment of motor speech disorders are several. First, assessments of motor speech disorders that assume a common pathophysiology for the limbs and the speech motor subsystems are likely to be in error. Further, the results reported in this paper pose serious problems in inferring from acoustical, aerodynamic, or perceptual observations to the pathophysiology of any particular subsystem. As was shown, the impaired movements of one structure are likely to influence the movements of a coupled structure and the subsystem-specific loci cannot be disambiguously identified without non-speech, physiological measures.

Finally, with regard to programs of rehabilitation, it appears that general approaches which assume a particular and common pathophysiology among speech and limb motor subsystems are, at best, likely to yield variable and uninterpretable results. At worst, such programs could actually exacerbate the control problem rather than ameliorating it. To illustrate this point, we should like to offer the physiological profile of a cerebral palsy individual diagnosed as a spastic dysarthric. One approach to spasticity has been muscle relaxation, thereby reducing the movement-induced reflexive muscle contractions that apparently interfere with normal movement patterns. Figure 2-17 shows the jaw and tongue force productions for this subject, using visual feedback, as with the records presented earlier.

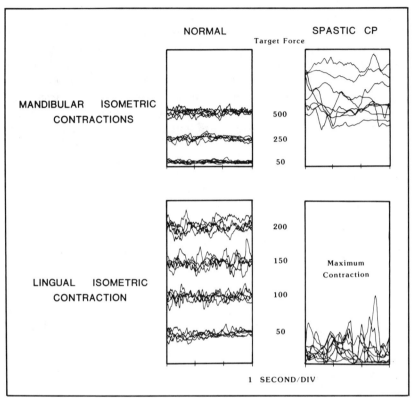

FIGURE 2-17
Comparison of mandibular and lingual force control in a normal subject and an adult spastic cerebral-palsied dysarthric subject.
*Notable is the inability by this dysarthric subject to produce lingual forces above 50 grams.

The jaw, as indicated previously, shows the classical signs of spasticity, i.e., an inability to produce low level stable forces, as might be required for fine speech control. However, the tongue shows a dramatically different impairment. Specifically, this subject was unable to produce any more than 15% of normal force, i.e., the tongue demonstrated substantial weakness. Indeed, based upon our analyses of labial biomechanics (Abbs and Muller, 1980), it would appear likely that this subject would have serious difficulty in producing normal closures for speech due to muscle weakness. The obvious point of this illustration is that if one had assumed uniform spasticity, and relaxation techniques had been employed, it is likely that the ability to produce adequate muscle contractions for speech in the tongue may have been exacerbated, albeit the jaw spasticity should have been somewhat relieved. This example, we believe, illustrates clearly the need to further develop assessment techniques for the evaluation of subsystem impairment that point more clearly to programs of focused differential subsystem rehabilitation and are tailored specifically to the nature of the involvement. Moreover, as evidenced in the case of the spastic cerebral-palsied individual with the bite-block (Figure 2-14), focused assessment yields information on the degree of impairment in different subcomponents; larger therapy gains are more likely to result if the most severe impairments are given initial and primary focus.

NOTE

[1]There remains a great deal of controversy concerning traditional descriptions of neurological disorders. As an example, accounts of Parkinsonism typically include resting tremor and cogwheeling among the characteristic symptomatology. Findley et al., (1981) have added action tremor, distinguishable from the other forms of involuntary activity in terms of frequency and characteristic EMG patterns, to the list of clinical features. Recent observations, such as these, tend to question the reliance upon classical limb descriptions to deductively identify the neuromuscular substrate of motor speech disorders. Further, the relationship between neuromuscular impairments and movement aberrations has not been clearly established. Evarts, Teravainen, and Calne (1981) found that the speed of response initiation and movement are independently impaired in Parkinson subjects. Despite systematic analysis, they were unable to attribute the characteristics symptoms; rigidity, tremor, to these movement impairments. Hence, the cause-effect relationship between volitional movement and underlying pathophysiology is not as straightforward as one is led to believe in traditional neurological texts.

REFERENCES

Abbs, J., & Eilenberg, G. Peripheral mechanisms of speech motor control. In N.J. Lass (Ed.), *Contemporary issues in experimental phonetics.* New York: Academic Press, 1976.

Abbs, J., & Muller, E. Neurophysiological and biomechanical factors in articulatory movement. Presented at the Conference on the Production of Speech, Austin TX, 1980.

Appenteng, K., O'Donovan, M., Somjen, G., Stephens, J., & Taylor, A. The projection of jaw elevator muscle spindle afferents to fifth nerve motoneurons in the cat. *Journal of Physiology*, 1978, *279*, 409-423.

Baken, R. Neuromuscular spindles in the intrinsic muscles of a human larynx. *Folia Phoniatricia*, 1971, *23*, 204-210.

Barlow, S., & Abbs, J. Force transducers for the evaluation of labial lingual and mandibular function in dysarthria. *Journal of Speech and Hearing Research,* in press.

Barlow, S., Cole, K., & Abbs, J. A new headmounted lip-jaw movement transduction system for the study of motor speech disorders. *Journal of Speech and Hearing Research,* in press.

Bowman, J., & Combs, C. The discharge pattern of lingual spindle afferent fibers in the hypoglottal nerve of the rhesus monkey. *Experimental Neurology,* 1968, *21,* 105.

Bratzlavsky, M., & vander Eecken, H. Afferent influences upon human genioglossal muscles. *Journal of Neurology,* 1974, *207,* 19-24.

Burke, R. Motor unit recruitment: What are the critical factors? J. Desmedt (Ed.), *New developments in electromyography and clinical neurophysiology.* Basel: Karger, 1981.

Canter, G. Speech characteristics of patients with Parkinson's disease: III articulation, diadochokinesis and overall speech adequacy. *Journal of Speech and Hearing Disorders,* 1963, *30,* 217-224.

Carpenter, M. *Human neuroanatomy.* Baltimore: Williams and Wilkins, 1976.

Cooper, S. Muscle spindles in the intrinsic muscles of the human tongue. *Journal of Physiology,* 1953, *122,* 193-202.

Darley, F., Aronson, A., & Brown, J. *Speech motor disorders.* Philadelphia: W.B. Saunders Co., 1975.

Darley, F., Aronson, A., & Brown, J. Differential diagnostic patterns of dysarthria. *Journal of Speech and Hearing Research,* 1969, *12,* 246-269. (a)

Darley F., Aronson, A., & Brown, J. Cluster of deviant speech dimension in the dysarthrias. *Journal of Speech and Hearing Research,* 1969, *12,* 462-496. (b)

Dubner, R., Sessle, B., & Storey, A. *The neural basis of oral and facial function.* New York: Plenum, 1978.

Evarts, E., Teravainen, H., & Calne, D. Reaction time in Parkinson's disease. *Brain*, 1981, *104*, 167-186.

Findley, L., Gresty, M. & Halmagyi, G. Tremor, the cogwheel phenomenon and clonus in Parkinson's disease. *Journal of Neurology, Neurosurgery and Psychiatry*, 1981, *44*, 534-546.

Fitzgerald, M., & Sachithanandan, S. The structure and source of lingual proprioceptors in the monkey. *Journal of Anatomy*, 1979, *128*, 523-552.

Folkins, J., & Larson, C. In search of a tonic vibration reflex in the human lip. *Brain Research*, 1978, *151*, 409-412.

Hardy, J. Development of neuromuscular systems underlying speech production. In *Speech and the dentofacial complex: The state of the art.* Proceeding of the workshop: ASHA Report 5. Washington, DC: American Speech and Hearing Association, 1970.

Harrison, F., & Corbin, K. The central pathway for the jaw-jerk. *American Journal of Physiology*, 1942, *135*, 439-445.

Henneman, E. Principles governing distribution of sensory input to motor neurons. In E. Evarts (Ed.), *Central Processing of sensory inputs leading to motor output.* Cambridge: MIT Press, 1975.

Henneman, E., Somjen, G., & Carpenter, D. Functional significance of cell size in spinal motorneurons. *Journal of Neurophysiology*, 1965, *28*, 560-580. (a)

Henneman, E., Somjen, G., & Carpenter, D. Excitibility and inhibitibility of motorneurons of different sizes. *Journal of Neurophysiology*, 1965, *28*, 599-620. (b)

Hixon, T. Respiratory-laryngeal evaluation. Presented at the Veterans Administration Workshop on Motor Speech Disorders, Madison, WS, 1975.

Hixon, T., & Hardy, J. Restricted mobility of the speech articulators in cerebral palsy. *Journal of Speech and Hearing Disorders*, 1964, *29*, 293-306.

Hixon, T., Goldman, M., & Mead, J. Kinematics of the chest wall during speech production. *Journal of Speech and Hearing Research,* 1973, *16,* 78-115.

Hixon, T., Mead, J., & Goldman, M. Dynamics of the chest wall during speech production: Function of the thorax, rib cage, diaphragm, and abdomen. *Journal of Speech and Hearing Research,* 1976, *19,* 297-356.

Holmes, G. Clinical symptoms of cerebellar diseases and their interpretations. The Croonian Lectures. *Lancet,* 1922, *100* (1), 1177-1182; *100* (2), 59-65, 111-115.

Houk, J. The physiology of muscle control configurations. In H. Drischel & P. Dettmer (Eds.), *The third international symposium on biocybernetics proceedings,* 1972.

Houk, J., & Rymer, W. Neural control of muscle length and tension. In V. Brooks (Ed.), *Motor control (handbook of physiology).* New York: Raven Press, 1981.

Hughes, O., & Abbs, J. Labial-mandibular coordination in the production of speech. *Phonetica,* 1976, *33,* 199-221.

Hunker, C., Abbs, J., & Barlow, S. The relationship between Parkinson rigidity and hypokinesia in the orofacial system: A quantitative analysis. *Neurology,* 1982, *32,* 749-756.

Hunker, C., Bless, D., & Weismer, G. Respiratory inductive plethysmography: A clinical technique for assuring respiratory function for speech. Paper presented at the meeting of the American Speech-Language-Hearing Association convention in Los Angeles, 1981.

Kent, R., & Netsell, R. A case study of an ataxic dysarthric: Cineradiographic and spectrographic observations. *Journal of Speech and Hearing Disorders,* 1975, *40,* 115-134.

Kent, R., & Netsell, R. Articulatory abnormalities in athetoid cerebral palsy. *Journal of Speech and Hearing Disorders,* 1978, *43,* 353-373.

Kent, R., & Netsell R. Acoustic-phonetic features of Parkinsonian dysarthria. Paper presented at the American Speech-Language-Hearing Association convention, Atlanta, 1979.

Kornhuber, H. Cerebral cortex, cerebellum, and basal ganglia: An introduction to their motor function. In E. Evarts (Ed.), *Central processing.* Cambridge: MIT Press, 1975.

Kubota, K., Masegi, T., & Osani, K. Muscle spindles in masticatory muscles and its trigimenal mesenciphalic nucleus. *Bulletin of the Tokyo Medical Dental University, 1974, 21.* (Supplement 3-6)

Kuypers, H. Corticobulbar connections to the pons and lower brainstem in man: An anatomical study. *Brain,* 1958, *81,* 364-388.

Larson, C., Sutton, D., & Lindeman, R. Muscle spindles in non-human primates laryngeal muscles. *Folia Prematologia,* 1974, *22,* 315-325.

Logemann, J., & Fisher, H. Vocal tract control in Parkinson's disease: Phonetic feature analysis of misarticulation. *Journal of Speech and Hearing Disorders,* 1981, *46,* 348-352.

Logemann, J., Fisher, H., Boshes, B., & Blonsky, B. Frequency and co-occurrence of vocal tract dysfunctions in speech of a large sample of Parkinsonian patients. *Journal of Speech and Hearing Disorders,* 1978, *43,* 47-57.

Lovell, M., Sutton, D., & Lindeman, R. Muscle spindles in non-human primates extrinsic auricular muscles. *Anatomical Review,* 1977, *189,* 519-524.

Lucas Keene, M. Muscle spindles in human laryngeal muscles. *Journal of Anatomy,* 1961, *95,* 25-29.

Lund, J., Richmond, F., Touloumis, C., Patry, Y., & Lamarre, Y. The distribution of ganglia tendon organs and muscle spindles in the masseter and temporalis muscles of the cat. *Neuroscience,* 1978, *3,* 259-270.

Milhorn, H. *The application of control theory to physiological systems.* Philadelphia: W. B. Saunders Co., 1966.

Muller, E., Abbs, J., & Kennedy, J. Some system physiology considerations for vocal control. In M. Hirano & K. Stevens (Eds.), *Proceedings of the conference on vocal fold physiology,* Kurume, Japan, 1980. University of Tokyo Press, 1981.

Neilson, P., Andrews, G., Guitar, B., & Quinn, P. Tonic stretch reflexes in lip, tongue, and jaw muscles. *Brain Research*, 1979, *178*, 311-327.

Netsell, R. A developing framework for research in speech production. Madison: Speech Research Laboratory, Neurological and Rehabilitation Hospital, University of Wisconsin, June 1971. (Progress report #1).

Netsell, R. Physiological studies of the dsyarthrias. Final progress report, NINCDS research grant 1971-1976, 1979.

Netsell, R., & Daniel, B. Dysarthria in adults: Physiological approach to rehabilitation. *Archives of Physical Medicine and Rehabilitation*, 1979, *60*, 502-508.

Partridge, L. A proposal for study of a static description of the motor control system. In M. Shahani (Ed.), *The motor system: Neurophysiological and muscle mechanics.* New York: Elsevier Scientific Publishing Co., 1976.

Patton, H., Sudsten, J., Crill, W., & Swanson, P. *Introduction to basic neurology.* Philadelphia: E.B. Saunders Co., 1976.

Penders, C., & Delwaide, P. Physiological approach to the human blink reflex. In J. Desmedt (Ed.), *New developments in electromyography and clinical neurophysiology.* Basel: Karger, 1973.

Robinson, D. The use of control systems analysis in neurophysiology of eye movements. *Annual Review of Neuroscience*, 1981, *4*, 463-503.

Rubow, R. Biofeedback in the treatment of speech disorders. Biofeedback Society of America Task Force Reports, 1981.

Rubow, R., & Flynn, M. Physiological biofeedback techniques in treatment of motor speech disorders. *Proceedings of the eleventh annual meeting of the Biofeedback Society of America.* Colorado Springs,

Rubow, R., & Netsell R. EMG biofeedback rehabilitation in facial paralysis: Ten year follow-up of a case study. *Proceedings of the tenth annual meeting of the Biofeedback Society of America.* San Diego, 1979.

Shahani, B., & Young, R. Blink reflexes in orbicularis oculi. In J. Desmedt (Ed.), *New developments in electromyography and clinical neurophysiology.* Basel: Karger, 1973.

Stein, R. What muscle variables does the nervous system control in limb movements. *The behavior and brain sciences,* in press.

Talbot, S., & Gessner, U. *Systems physiology.* New York: John Wiley and Sons, 1973.

Watson, C. Functional deficits and the patterns of degeneration following lesions of the face motor cortex in the Macaca Mulatta. *Anatomical Review,* 1973, *175,* 465.

ACKNOWLEDGEMENT

This work was supported in part by NINCDS Program Grant NS-13274-05.

3

Suprasegmental and Prosodic Considerations in Motor Speech Disorders

Gary J. Barnes

INTRODUCTION

In the days when dysarthria was defined as "slurred speech," the study of suprasegmentals and prosodic features in speech production remained primarily within the province of linguistics. Remediation was focused at the segmental levels as clinicians meticulously directed articulation drills, plodding systematically from phoneme to phoneme. Although Monrad-Krohn (1947) presented one of the earliest descriptions of a prosodic disturbance in a neurologically impaired patient, it was not until after the middle 1950s and early 1960s that this knowledge was applied to motor speech disorders. During this time, phoneticians and speech scientists began to posit acoustic descriptions of suprasegmentals and prosodic features. Darley, Aronson, and Brown (1969 a and b) in their classic perceptual study of the dysarthrias, described them in terms of deviant perceptual dimensions of speech. Among the 38 dimensions they studied were 10 dimensions they labeled as prosodic deviations.

Subsequent clinicians have continued to report the disturbance of suprasegmentals and prosodic features in motor speech disorders. These symptoms have refused to go away even as we did our best to ignore them.

It has been stated that these disturbances exist in the speech patterns of all dysarthric individuals (Rosenbek and LaPointe, 1978). With regard to apraxia of speech, prosodic disturbances are considered to be one of the defining characteristics of this controversial disorder, which has been described succinctly as a sensorimotor disorder of articulation and prosody (Rosenbek, 1978). Given the significant contribution of suprasegmental and prosodic disturbances to the symptom complex of motor speech disorders, one might expect a surplus of research findings from which to construct bases for treatment techniques. Unfortunately, this has not occurred. With the exception of continued statements, most often based on perceptual data, that, indeed, something is amiss with the melodic line of speech, there has been a paucity of research designed to document the acoustic characteristics and physiological constructs of prosody in disordered speech production. Rosenbek (1978) surmised that perhaps at one time the suprasegmentals and prosodic features were considered to be the "formal wear" of speech production and, as such, "could be done without" (p. 219). Another viewpoint held that suprasegmentals and prosodic features were entirely dependent and subject to intact segmental production. This may have relegated the study of these disturbances to a "holding tank" while researchers focused on the constructs of segmental production, in the hope that their findings could explain and account for the perceived prosodic disturbances.

Currently, these viewpoints are of only historical interest. An entire session at the recent Clinical Dysarthria Conference was devoted to the topic of Prosody, which is reflective of the recent efforts of investigators to provide acoustic and physiological descriptions of prosodic features in motor speech disorders. Accompanying this descriptive research are efforts designed to evaluate treatment methodologies for prosodic disturbances.

My purpose in this presentation is to provide an up-to-date view of the relationship of suprasegmental and prosodic considerations to motor speech disorders. This review will focus on various issues of speech prosody such as confusions pertaining to terminology, methodological considerations in assessment, as well as a review of the studies that have included suprasegmentals and prosodic features as variables of interest in the study of individuals with a motor speech disorder.

DEFINITIONS:
WHAT A TANGLED WEB WE WEAVE . . .

Hamlet's statement aptly describes the literature that has attempted to provide definitions of relevant terminology. The study of suprasegmentals and prosodic features is not lacking in descriptive terms, but is lacking in agreed-upon definitions of these terms. Prominence, pitch accent, force, emphasis, intonation, breath-group, accent-up, accent-down, stress, rhythm, tempo, tone, and juncture are but a few of the terms which confront the reader of this literature. A review of the classic studies of these features in normal speech production, such as work of Fry (1955, 1958), Bolinger (1955, 1958), Lieberman (1967, 1970) and Lehiste (1970), indicates that although the terminology is different, the underlying acoustic patterns are relatively similar. Hence, many of the terms become interchangeable.

One confusion in the literature pertains to relationship between the terms "suprasegmental" and "prosodic." Although often used synonymously in the literature, current researchers have attempted to delineate differences between the terms. Rosenbek and LaPointe (1978) stated that the suprasegmentals include pitch, loudness, articulation time, and pause time. They define prosodic features as those features that are produced by the interaction of the suprasegmentals. Definitions were provided for three prosodic features: rhythm, stress, and intonation. Their definition of the suprasegmentals is in general agreement with Lehiste, however, Lehiste does not refer to rhythm, stress, and intonation as prosodic features. She suggests that rhythm, stress, and intonation represent the linguistic function of the suprasegmentals operating at the sentence level. Crystal (1969), while agreeing that prosodic features result from variations in pitch, loudness, and duration, either in isolation or combination, does not refer to pitch, loudness, and duration as suprasegmentals. He refers to them as "attributes" of speech. Clearly, the different is in terminology as there is good agreement on the existence of the phenomena. Specifically, there is agreement that certain effects (prosodic features? linguistic functions?) are realized across speech segments by the interaction of pitch, loudness, articulation time, and pause time (attributes? suprasegmentals?).

Rosenbek and LaPointe (1978) proposed the following clinical basis for the distinction between suprasegmentals and prosodic features. They stated that certain "patterns of error in the dysarthrias, such as inadequate loudness in a patient with essentially normal pitch, articulation time, pause time, stress, and intonation, lead us to the distinction" (p. 299). In the instance just described, the deficit in what they refer to as a suprasegmental (loudness) did not result in a disturbance of a prosodic feature (stress). Clinical data, collected in a systematic manner, may indicate whether this distinction is real and/or relevant. In this presentation I will refer to rhythm, stress, and intonation as prosodic features that are the result of interaction among pitch, loudness, articulation time, and pause time. The term "suprasegmental" will be used in the clinical context described by Rosenbek and LaPointe. However, the study of prosodic features will be of primary interest.

Netsell (1973) provided operational definitions of the three prosodic features. *Rhythm* was defined as "the perception of the time program applied to the phonetic events" (p. 224). The durational relationship between pause time and articulation time is the suprasegmental feature primarily responsible for the perceived prosodic feature of rhythm. The second prosodic feature, referred to as *stress*, was defined by Netsell as "the perception of syllable emphasis, relative to the emphasis perceived on other syllables in the same sentence, or phrase" (p. 224). The prosodic feature of stress is not as amenable to description by a single acoustic parameter. The perceived emphasis (defined in much of the literature as "prominence") that occurs when a syllable is stressed may result from fundamental frequency shifts, durational changes, intensity variations, spectral changes in the vowels, or any combination of the parameters. The contribution of each of these parameters to the prosodic feature of stress is variable both between and within speakers. Brain damage may serve to restrict the range of combinations that will result in perceived stress differences.

The last prosodic feature to be defined is *intonation*. Netsell defined this as "the perception of changes in the fundamental frequency of vocal fold vibration (f_0) during speech production" (p. 224). The suprasegmental most closely related to this prosodic feature is pitch. Studies of intonation patterns in brain-damaged individuals have investigated variables such as terminal contour, pitch range, pitch changes over time, and pitch direction (Keatley, 1975; Danly, de Villiers, and Cooper, 1979).

METHODOLOGICAL CONSIDERATIONS

In the assessment of the prosodic features in motor speech disorders, the clinician must make judgments of rhythm, stress, and intonation. Questions of rhythm might include: Is the rate appropriate? If not, is articulation time or pause time, or both, inappropriate? When considering stress: Is stress being achieved on the right syllables? Is stress observable at both the word and sentence level? How is stress being achieved? Finally, the questions of intonation: Are pitch changes appropriate? Can the patient achieve a variety of intonation contours? Focusing on the suprasegmentals of pitch and loudness, the clinician must decide if the overall range and levels are appropriate.

The methods for assessment of suprasegmental and prosodic disturbances are relatively few and can be characterized as either perceptual or acoustic in nature. Using primarily perceptual means, certain suprasegmentals can be investigated in isolation. For example, the patient's pitch and loudness, which are dependent primarily on the laryngeal and respiratory systems respectively, can be studied independently, to a degree. Certainly, fundamental frequency and intensity, the acoustic correlates of pitch and loudness, can be measured as well.

Perceptual measures of the prosodic features of stress, rhythm, and intonation have provided general information, at best. One example of a perceptual judgment is the assessment of melodic line as one component of the rating scale of speech characteristics, part of the *Boston Diagnostic Aphasia Examination* (Goodglass and Kaplan, 1972). As defined on the test form, melodic line corresponds to the prosodic feature of intonation. Keatley (1975) suggested that an assessment of intonation should include the production of Yes/No questions ("Is it there?") which appear to be sensitive to prosodic disturbances.

Contrastive stress drills have been proposed as one method for the perceptual assessment of stress and rhythm (Rosenbek and LaPointe, 1978). These drills, adapted from exercises for vocal prominence by Fairbanks (1960), provide a structured task for obtaining a perceptual assessment of phrase level stress. For example, the patient may be instructed to say the sentence "Pat paid Bob." The clinician would then ask questions that would require the patient to stress one of the words to convey the appropriate meaning. Questions might include: "Who paid Bob?" "Pat paid who?" "Did Pat hit Bob?" One advantage of this method over observations of spontaneous speech is the ability of the clinician to control for both length and phonetic context, which minimizes the effect of inadequate articulation on the prosodic feature of stress. A possible disadvantage may be the limited inference of the patient's speaking behavior in contrastive stress drills to other tasks requiring prosodic manipulations. For example, a contrastive stress drill comprised of single-syllable words may by more sensitive to a general increase in speaker effort than tasks such as the distinction between production of noun-verb stress pairs (as in 'record and re'cord) which may require more subtle manipulations of the acoustic parameters of stress.

Further specification of suprasegmental and prosodic variables has resulted from acoustic analysis of the speech patterns of individuals with motor speech disorders. The primary method of acoustic analysis in motor speech disorders has been spectrographic analysis. Examples of this application can be found in studies by Kent and Netsell (1975) and Kent, Netsell, and Abbs (1979), who investigated parameters such as voice-onset time (VOT), duration, and intonation patterns in ataxic dysarthric individuals. Kent and Rosenbek (in press) will report spectrographic data on apraxic speakers, hypokinetic dysarthrics, and right-hemisphere lesion patients, in addition to the data on ataxic dysarthrics.

Computer analysis was employed in the acoustic investigation of ataxic dysarthria in a study by Yorkston and Beukelman (1981). Data were reported for the acoustic parameters of fundamental frequency, duration, and relative intensity levels. Danly et al. (1979) employed similar computerized techniques to assess aspects of fundamental frequency contours as well as segmental timing.

The results of such acoustic studies hold great promise for clinicians interested in both the acoustic documentation of perceptual symptoms and the development of treatment techniques.

REVIEW OF PERTINENT STUDIES

Unfortunately, only a handful of studies have included suprasegmentals and/or prosodic features as variables of interest. Of the dysarthrias, ataxic dysarthria has been the primary object of prosodic research, although hypokinetic dysarthria has also been defined acoustically in terms. of prosodic considerations.

The primary acoustic studies of ataxic dysarthria are those by Kent and his colleagues (Kent and Netsell, 1975; Kent, Netsell, and Abbs, 1979). The earlier study reported both physiological and acoustic data, cineradiographic and spectrographic data respectively, in one individual with ataxic dysarthria (Kent and Netsell, 1975). The acoustic characteristics identified in this subject included long segment durations, and monotone patterns with occasional "marked and inappropriate changes in the fundamental frequency" (p. 127). The subsequent study (Kent, Netsell, and Abbs, 1979) provided similar acoustic data on five additional ataxic dysarthrics. Their speech was recorded in a variety of stimulus, conditions, including a comparison of structured versus spontaneous speech, and then analyzed spectrographically. The results from this investigation were consistent with the original case study in 1975, namely, that ataxic dysarthria is characterized by lengthening of segments in atypical proportion, which disrupts the normal timing of speech patterns. In addition, other characteristics included wide and periodic intervals between syllables and generally flat fundamental frequency (F_0) contours with occasional instances of inappropriate F_0 changes. The two studies taken together provide evidence that correlates the acoustic data with the perceptual data provided by Brown, Darley, and Aronson (1970), who presented a comprehensive perceptual analysis of ataxic dysarthria.

Additional acoustic evidence of disrupted prosodic features in ataxic dysarthria was provided by Yorkston and Beukelman (1981). They described the patterns of fundamental frequency contour, relative intensity, and duration in an ataxic individual attempting to produce contrastive stress. They reported that this individual had only durational constraints available to signal stress, since he had limited control of fundamental frequency and intensity levels. Attempts to use pitch and loudness to signal stress resulted in what they described as "bizarreness with sweeping changes in fundamental frequency and extreme bursts of intensity" (p. 402). The disruption of the suprasegmentals, pitch and loudness, is reflected in the disrupted prosodic feature of stress. As the acoustic data indicate, all of the prosodic features (rhythm, stress, and intonation) are ravaged in ataxic dysarthria. This is not particularly surprising given the degree of coordination required for the production of prosodic features in speech, and the nature of the deficit in ataxic dysarthria.

In addition to ataxic dysarthria, Kent and Rosenbek's study will provide an acoustic description of selected parameters in hypokinetic dysarthria, which may account for the prosodic disturbances perceived in some individuals with Parkinson's disease. Darley et al. (1969) reported that the hypokinetic dysarthria observed in Parkinson patients consisted of a group of deviant speech dimensions, among which was a correlated subgroup they referred to collectively as a cluster of prosodic insufficiency Kent and Rosenbek (in press) will report that this pattern can be observed spectrographically as a general reduction in acoustic detail. Although the particular acoustic characteristics may vary among Parkinson patients, the effect on prosody is generally one of attenuation of the normal prosodic patterns.

A similar effect on prosody has been observed in a few individuals with right-hemisphere cortical lesions. Kent and Rosenbek will provide spectrographic data which is remarkably similar to the acoustic patterns observed in hypokinetic dysarthria. Prominent among the similarities is a "tendency toward monotone, indistinct articulation, and mild to moderate hypernasality" (p. 28, original manuscript), which is reflected in the spectrograms as reduced acoustic detail and a reduction of energy in the mid-frequency region. The need for continued research into the nature of the acoustic similarities between these two distinct neuropathologies is apparent.

Study of the prosodic disturbance in apraxia of speech has been rather limited, especially when compared to ataxic dysarthria. Early definitions of apraxia of speech considered prosodic disturbances to be the logical result of compensation for an articulatory disorder. More recent definitions have suggested that prosodic disturbances may be a primary characteristic of the disorder, and not simply a secondary symptom to disrupted articulation. Even with the emphasis on prosody as a critical variable to be considered in diagnosis, there have been only limited efforts to document the acoustic characteristics of apraxia of speech.

In the same discussion of prosodic disturbance and neurogenic lesion, Kent and Rosenbek will present spectrographic data on the speech patterns of seven apraxic speakers. They will report that the primary characteristic of reduced rate is due to at least two processes, articulatory prolongation and syllable segregation. Articulatory prolongation is observed as an increase in the length of steady-states or transitions within a speech pattern, resulting in considerably longer durations than normal. Syllable segregation is observed as lengthened pause time between consecutive syllables. They further state that the apraxic demonstrates "a speech pattern that is perceived as halting (especially because of segment prolongations and inappropriate pauses), occasionally phonetically inaccurate (for example, the voicing errors), and abnormally stressed (particularly because of a general tendency toward segment prolongation and a failure to effect syllable reduction when appropriate)" (p. 18-19, original manuscript).

Although in the most severe cases there may be a few intonation contours extending across syllables, both Danly et al. (1979) and Gelfer (1980) reported that their apraxic speakers appeared to retain certain aspects of speech prosody. Danly et al. reported that two aspects of fundamental frequency contours (terminal falling f_0 contour and declination of f_0 peaks) were evident in both spontaneous speech and oral reading tasks. In contrast, Keatley (1975) reported data on intonational contours in apraxia of speech which demonstrated that apraxic subjects may have a restricted pitch range, may not raise pitch at the appropriate times, and may demonstrate minimal pitch changes in the terminal contour. Finally, Gelfer (1980) indicated that, on an inconsistent basis, her apraxic subject was able to achieve stress on targeted syllables by manipulating the parameters of frequency, intensity, and duration. As in ataxic dysarthria, the prosodic feature most disrupted in apraxia of speech is the rhythm, or timing, of speech patterns.

SUPRASEGMENTALS AND PROSODIC FEATURES
AS TREATMENT VARIABLES

Although prosodic disturbances, such as those just described, have been identified as primary characteristics in motor speech disorders, there have been few investigations of prosodic features as treatment variables. Previously, treatment of prosodic features occurred late, if at all, in a treatment program. However, current investigators have proposed that the treatment of prosodic features should constitute a major focus of attention. (Rosenbek, 1978; Yorkston and Beukelman, 1981). It has been suggested that the treatment of prosodic features may have a facilitory effect on segmental production, although controlled study of this clinical intuition is yet to be done. One source for this speculation was a study by Kent and Netsell (1972), which investigated the effect of stress contrasts on articulation in a few normal subjects. One effect of stress was to increase articulatory accuracy.

The prosodic feature of rhythm has received the most attention in the treatment literature. The age-old clinical adage "Slow down" is but one example. The process of rate control has been cited as essential to achieving maximal intelligibility in individuals with a motor speech disorder. The clinical application of one form of rate control, referred to as *pacing,* was described by Nailling and Horner (1979). They suggested that imposed pacing strategies may improve intelligibility in certain individuals with either apraxia of speech, ataxic dysarthria, mixed ataxic-spastic dysarthria, or spastic dysarthria. One effect of many rate control strategies is to regulate rhythm, many times producing equalized stress patterns which differ from the normal prosodic patterns of speech. The critical task of the clinician is to work towards normal prosodic patterns while, at the same time, not sacrificing the gains in intelligibility achieved by rate control strategies. A successful example of this task was reported by Yorkston and Beukelman (1981). They suggested that once rate control has been achieved by the patient, less rigid and more appropriate cueing techniques may be utilized. In addition, they report success in training strategies for achieving normalized stress patterns, based on an individual's control of particular suprasegmental features. Three of their four subjects were trained to manipulate durational variables, while the fourth subject utilized an intensity adjustment to signal stress.

Additional information on the treatment of prosodic features in motor speech disorders was provided by Rosenbek and LaPointe (1978). They provided suggestions for the modification of the individual suprasegmentals as well as the treatment of the prosodic features. Contrastive stress drills were recommended as one method for presentation of stimuli for treatment tasks.

A review of the clinical literature suggests that techniques such as pacing and other rate control strategies are not new. Further treatment techniques for prosodic disturbances may not need to be new; perhaps the effects of current treatment techniques in dysarthria should be studied and recognized for their effect on prosody. Although in its infancy, the systematic study of the treatment of prosodic variables in motor speech disorders is encouraging.

CONCLUDING REMARKS

Naturally, many questions and concerns of importance remain to be addressed. Foremost among these concerns is the relationship of the observed prosodic disturbances in various motor speech disorders to the underlying neural structures and processsess. Based on acoustic and perceptual observations of the prosodic disturbances in apraxia of speech, ataxic dysarthria, hypokinetic dysarthria, and the speech patterns of right-hemisphere patients. Kent and Rosenbek (in press) will propose hypotheses pertaining to the production of prosodic features and their neurological substrates.

Further study of the acoustical characteristics of prosodic features in motor speech disorders may answer a few questions, but will probably create more. However, bits and pieces of information, gleaned from controlled investigations, will eventually result in a systematic methodology for the improvement of prosodic features in individuals with a motor speech disorder.

REFERENCES

Bolinger, D. Intersections of stress and intonation. *Word, 1955, 11,* 195-203.

Bolinger, D. A theory of pitch accent in English. *Word, 1958, 14,* 109-149.

Brown, J., Darley, F., & Aronson, A. Ataxic dysarthria. *International Journal of Neurology,* 1970, 7, 302-318.

Crystal, D. *Prosodic systems and intonation in English.* Cambridge, England: Cambridge University Press, 1969.

Danly, M., deVilliers, J., & Cooper, W. Control of speech prosody in Broca's aphasia. Paper presented to the Acoustical Society of America. Cambridge, MA, 1979.

Darley, F., Aronson, A., & Brown, J. Differential diagnostic patterns of dysarthria. *Journal of Speech and Hearing Research,* 1969, *12,* 246-269. (a)

Darley, F., Aronson, A., & Brown, J. Clusters of deviant speech dimensions in the dysarthrias. *Journal of Speech and Hearing Research,* 1969, *12,* 462-496. (b)

Fairbanks, G. *Voice and articulation drillbook.* New York: Harper & Row, 1960.

Fry, D. Duration and intensity as physical correlates of linguistic stress. *Journal of the Acoustical Society of America,* 1955, *27,* 765-768.

Fry, D. Experiments in the perception of stress. *Language and Speech,* 1958, *1,* 126-152.

Gelfer, C. The ability to vary stress in a subject with apraxia of speech. Paper presented to the Acoustical Society of America, Atlanta, GA, 1980.

Goodglass, H., & Kaplan, E. *The assessment of aphasia and related disorders.* Philadelphia: Lea & Febiger, 1972.

Keatley, M. Intonational contours in apraxia of speech. Unpublished master's thesis, University of Colorado, 1975.

Kent, R., & Netsell, R. Effects of stress contrasts on certain articulatory parameters. *Phonetica,* 1972, *24,* 23-24.

Kent, R., & Netsell, R. A case study of an ataxic dysarthria: Cineradiographic and spectrographic observations. *Journal of Speech and Hearing Disorders,* 1975, *40,* 115-134.

Kent, R., & Rosenbek, J. Prosodic disturbance and neurogenic lesion. *Brain and Language,* in press.

Kent, R., Netsell, R., & Abbs, J. Acoustic characteristics of dysarthria associated with cerebellar disease. *Journal of Speech and Hearing Research*, 1972, *22*, 627-648.

Lehiste, I. *Suprasegmentals.* Cambridge: MIT Press, 1970.

Lieberman, P. *Intonation, perception and language,* Cambridge: MIT Press, 1967.

Lieberman, P. A study of prosodic features. *Haskins Lab. Status Rep. Sp. Res. SR-23*, 1970, 179-208.

Monrad-Krohn, G. Dysprosody or altered 'melody of language.' *Brain*, 1947, *70*, 405-415.

Nailling, K., & Horner, J. Reorganizing neurogenic articulation disorders by modifying prosody. Paper presented at the convention of the American Speech-Language-Hearing Association, Atlanta, 1979.

Netsell, R. Speech physiology. In F. Minifie, T. Hixon, & F. Williams (Eds.), *Normal aspects of speech, hearing and language.* Englewood Cliffs, NJ: Prentice-Hall, 1973.

Rosenbek, J. Treating apraxia of speech. In D.F. Johns (Ed.), *Clinical management of neurogenic communicative disorders.* Boston: Little, Brown and Co., 1978.

Rosenbek, J., & LaPointe, L. The dysarthrias: Description, diagnosis, and treatment. In D. Johns (Ed.), *Clinical management of neurogenic communicative disorders.* Boston: Little, Brown and Co., 1978.

Yorkston, K., & Beukelman, D. Ataxic dysarthria: Treatment sequences based on intelligibility and prosodic considerations. *Journal of Speech and Hearing Disorders,* 1981, *46*, 398-404.

ACKNOWLEDGMENTS

The author wishes to thank Albyn Davis and Steve Harmon for their helpful comments, criticisms, and suggestions during the preparation of this manuscript.

4

The Production of Stress in Three Types of Dysarthric Speech

Thomas Murry

INTRODUCTION

The information in the speech signal can be imparted in one of two ways, either by the words chosen or by the manner in which the words are produced. The second requires the talker to make use of the suprasegmental or prosodic features of a language. In order to show the importance of a syllable or word, that word or syllable is stressed. Stress is traditionally defined as an abstract entity generated by phonological rules indicating the relative importance of different syllables and usually reflected by a greater degree of articulatory effort (Rabiner, Levitt, and Rosenberg, 1969; Lieberman, 1967). Synonymous with stress in spoken language are the terms *emphasis, prominence, importance, and significance.*

In normal speech, stress is most commonly produced by an increase in fundamental frequency, intensity, duration, and articulatory effort (Fry, 1955). Other features such as juncture and the reduction of an adjacent word or syllable may also be utilized to indicate stress. Usually, no single prosodic feature is used to produce the stress; rather a combination of features is used. Consider the phrase, *BOB BIT TODD.* for the word *bit,* the stress will usually be produced with a combination of increased fundamental frequency and intensity since the vowel is lax and, according to the phonological rules of English, lax vowels are not lengthened significantly in stressed versus unstressed syllables. In vowels such as /ɑ/ or /i/, duration would be increased along with frequency and intensity in a stressed relative to an unstressed syllable. The production of appropriate stress in normal speech requires intact respiratory, phonatory, and articulatory systems.

The inability to produce adequate stress in speech is characteristic of many types of dysarthria. Dysarthric speech consists of distortions relating not only to the words chosen to produce the speech but also to the suprasegmentals used to impart meaning. This could be heard in the monotone voice of the Parkinsonian patient or the stacatto-like speech of the ataxic patient, in which each syllable appears to have equal emphasis, a fact which has been documented in at least one investigation (Kent, Netsell, and Abbs, 1979).

The information that exists to describe the stress patterns of dysarthric speech stems mainly from the perceptual investigations done at the Mayo Clinic, using relatively large numbers of subjects and the skills of clinicians familiar with dysarthric speech. Other studies that have used fewer subjects have provided corroborative information about the perceptual features identified by the Mayo group. Only recently have investigators turned their attention to quantifying the features of dysarthria that in the past have shown perceptual relevance (Yorkston, Beukelman, and Minifie, 1979). These studies, which have been reviewed by Barnes (1983), suggest that quantification of the speech and voice parameters of the dysarthrias contributes to the diagnosis and treatment of these problems. The purpose of the present investigation is to examine the manner in which dysarthric speakers use physiologic and acoustic features to impart stress to a one-syllable word. Perceptually, it has been shown that certain types of dysarthria are more deviant in dimensions that relate to stress. For example, consider the data from Darley, Aronson, and Brown (1975) shown in Table 4-1. In the first column, five features relating to stress are listed and the rank and perceptual scale value assigned to that group follow.

It may be presumed from the table that hypokinetic patients are perceived to have the most abnormal stress since they rate high on ratings of monopitch and monoloudness. Loudness and pitch are two of the three most significant contributors to perceived stress. The spastic and ataxic groups, who also have highly ranked scale values for these features, would be expected to have stress deviations, but not as severe as the hypokinetic. The perceptual data in Table 4-1 provide the point of departure for this investigation. This study presents an acoustic and physiologic analysis of the features which contribute to spoken stress in dysarthric speech.

TABLE 4-1
Rank order and mean scale values of five stress-related perceptual features in three types of dysarthria.

Dimension	SPASTIC		ATAXIC		HYPOKINETIC	
	Rank	Mean Scale Value	Rank	Mean Scale Value	Rank	Mean Scale Value
Monopitch	2	3.72	8	1.74	1	4.64
Monoloudness	5	2.98	9	1.62	3	4.26
Reduced Stress	3	3.32		*	2	4.46
Excess/ Equal Stress	14	1.50	2	2.69		*
Slow Rate	7	-2.66	10	-1.59		*

*No significant scale value

METHOD

Subjects

Fourteen dysarthric subjects were selected for this study after examining the records of approximately 35 dysarthric patients. A normal group of five subjects was selected from a group of volunteers. Table 4-2 presents the breakdown of the four groups.

There were five subjects in the normal, spastic, and ataxic groups; four subjects were studied from the hypokinetic group. All subjects were males. The age range was 30-70 years. No attempt was made to match groups. The only criteria utilized to select the subjects was a confirming diagnosis by a neurologist, a relatively stable neurologic condition, the ability to perform the tasks, and no treatment prior to the testing date.

Type		Age	Etiology	Months Post Onset
TABLE 4-2				
List of subjects included in this study.				
Normal	N1	38		
	N2	27		
	N3	26		
	N4	44		
	N5	32		
Spastic	S1	33	Motor Vehicle Accident	11
	S2	61	CVA	1
	S3	52	CVA	61
	S4	56	L. CVA	2
	S5	74	Bilat. CVA	72
Ataxic	A1	69	CVA	3
	A2	52	Multiple Sclerosis	60
	A3	58	CVA	3
	A4	69	Progressive Cerebellar Degen.	12
	A5	60	Multiple Sclerosis	12
Hypokinetic	H1	55	Parkinson's	300
	H2	74	Parkinson's	24
	H3	68	Parkinson's	84
	H4	62	Shy-Drager Syndrome	?

Equipment

Figure 4-1 shows a block diagram of the experimental apparatus. The subject was seated in front of a differential pressure transducer. A polyethylene tube was inserted in his mouth to fit behind the point of consonant articulation. The pressure signal was transduced to an amplifier and recorded on a light writing oscillograph (Honeywell 1508 C). A tape recorder was positioned nearby to record the acoustic signal. From the polyethylene tube, intraoral air pressure associated with consonant production was recorded. From the tape recorder, the acoustic measures were derived.

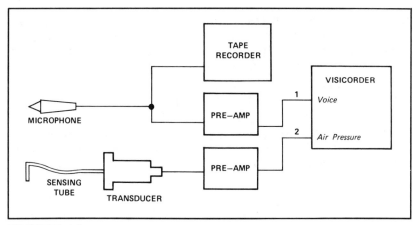

FIGURE 4-1
Block diagram of the recording apparatus used to obtain the five prosodic measures

Procedures

Each subject produced twenty repetitions of the phrase *BOB BIT TODD*. He was instructed to say the sentence once as he normally spoke it. Then he was asked three questions: "Who bit Bob?" "Did Bob kick Todd?" and "Did Bob bite Sam?" The same sentence was never repeated twice in succession. Thus, there were five sentences spoken in the normal manner, five with intended stress on *Bob*, five with intended stress on *bit* and five with intended stress on *Todd*. The first five sentences served as the baseline set and all comparisons were made with the words in the baseline sentence.

Measurement and Analysis

Five measures of stress were obtained and analyzed: peak intraoral pressure, integrated pressure-time, fundamental frequency, vowel duration, and vowel intensity. The first two were taken for the consonant, either /b/ or /t/; the final three from the vowel /ɑ/. The word *bit* was not analyzed in this study.

The peak intraoral air pressure was measured in centimeters of water and considered to be the highest point in the pressure pulse associated with consonant articulation. Integrated pressure-time was obtained by plotting the time course of the pressure pulse from its baseline departure through the peak and back to the baseline. It is plotted with a compensating polar planimeter and measured in centimeters of water per second. Detailed methods for obtaining the two measures have been presented by Brown and McGlone (1974), Murry and Brown (1976), Brown and Shearer (1970), and Muller and Brown (1980).

The three acoustic measures, frequency, intensity, and duration were obtained from the vocalic portions of the words *Bob* and *Todd*. The vocalic portions were identified from the visicorder tracings. The fundamental frequency was obtained from one channel of the visicorder output by counting the number of cycles in the vocalic portion. These portions were identified as the continuous voicing segments between the two plosive bursts. When the volume was low, the time-locked pressure pulse from the other channel of the visicorder helped to determine the vocalic portion.

Duration was obtained from the same vocalic portion of the visicorder trace used to identify fundamental frequency. The duration of the vocalic portion was measured in millimeters and converted to milliseconds.

All measures of intensity of the stressed syllable were made relative to the baseline values. In order to obtain a measure of intensity, the original tape recordings were recorded onto one channel of a two-channel audio recorder. On the second channel, a 70 dB HL pure tone from an audiometer set to O VU was recorded. The output of the two channels was directed to a two-channel storage oscilloscope. The vertical scale of the oscilloscope was set to ten divisions for the 70 dB pure tone. The number of vertical divisions for the vowel on channel two were counted. Thus, all intensity measures were relative to the 70 dB HL 125 Hz pure tone. A measure of intensity units was obtained by dividing the final values by a constant obtained from the oscilloscope amplification.

For each subject, five measures of stress were obtained for five productions of *Bob* and five productions of *Todd*. The two consonant-related measures of air pressure and the three vowel-related measures of frequency, duration, and intensity in the stressed syllables were compared to those measures in the unstressed syllables.

RESULTS

Table 4-3 shows the results of five measures of stress for each of the groups for the words *Bob* and *Todd*.

TABLE 4-3
Mean and standard deviation of the measures of stress for the words *Bob* and *Todd* for each group of talkers.

		P_0 cm H_2O		P_{10} cm H_2O/sec		f_0 Hz		DUR (msec)		INT (units)	
		X	SD	X	SD	X	SD	X	SD	X	SD
BOB											
Normals	ST	4.6	2.5	.47	.47	131.8	22.4	198.6	23.7	13.1	3.2
	UNST	2.9	1.5	.25	.19	108.2	22.8	180.7	21.2	9.9	2.7
Spastic	ST	5.3	3.1	.66	.48	133.3	31.1	256.5	54.3	9.9	2.6
	UNST	4.0	3.8	.47	.56	129.1	32.6	263.5	65.4	9.3	2.1
Ataxic	ST	6.9	3.8	.80	.56	130.3	22.6	249.0	113.0	11.9	2.8
	UNST	5.6	2.8	.65	.36	124.4	26.3	269.3	115.0	11.3	2.1
Hypokinetic	ST	2.2	1.1	.23	.10	148.5	39.4	168.1	42.1	10.0	5.7
	UNST	2.3	1.4	.25	.15	143.2	29.7	164.3	33.6	9.6	6.5
TODD											
Normals	ST	6.8	1.9	.54	.43	116.1	5.9	291.7	77.2	10.0	3.0
	UNST	5.9	1.2	.41	.32	96.5	14.2	262.6	88.5	8.2	2.3
Spastic	ST	10.5	8.6	2.45	3.02	136.1	36.8	270.6	105.4	8.8	1.7
	UNST	10.5	9.4	3.53	4.01	126.5	33.6	284.4	115.0	8.0	1.8
Ataxic	ST	9.2	3.6	1.28	.59	123.9	22.1	301.3	86.6	10.0	2.8
	UNST	10.3	3.7	1.69	.75	113.8	24.3	281.7	78.5	8.3	2.5
Hypokinetic	ST	7.8	6.4	2.78	2.22	127.4	24.7	348.4	100.4	9.1	4.9
	UNST	8.4	6.6	1.40	1.55	126.8	28.5	344.8	112.2	8.9	5.6

The stress pattern for the normal subjects shows the values greater in the stressed than the unstressed conditions for all measures for both words. The normal subjects produced air pressure and integrated pressure-time values for /t/ that exceeded those for /b/. Fundamental frequency and intensity are higher in the initial word position than the final. The vowel duration is longer in the final than in the initial position. Thus, the normal subjects show a stressed/unstressed difference for all measures. In addition, they show a word-order effect in which the absolute values are generally greater in the initial position.

The air pressure patterns for the spastic and ataxic groups are similar to the normal group for *Bob*, but not *Todd*. The spastic group showed relatively no difference in the three acoustic measures for *Bob*. This group accomplished initial word stress by increasing pressure and integrated pressure-time. For final word stress, the spastic group used only fundamental frequency to impart stress. The ataxic group used both air pressure parameters to stress the word *Bob*, and fundamental frequency, duration, and intensity to stress *Todd*. The hypokinetic group did not use any of the five measures to produce a stressed/unstressed difference in the production of the two words. Their values indicate that they reduced pressure and changed the vowel parameters very little from the stressed to unstressed words.

The data of Table 4-3 were subjected to an analysis of variance. Main effect differences of stress and word, and the group-by-stress interaction were significant at the .05 level. The data in Table 4-3 suggest that the normal subjects differ from the three neuropathological groups and the hypokinetic group differs from the spastic and ataxic groups in the way they impart word stress. The spastic and ataxic groups did not differ significantly from each other for any measure of word stress with the exception of integrated pressure-time.

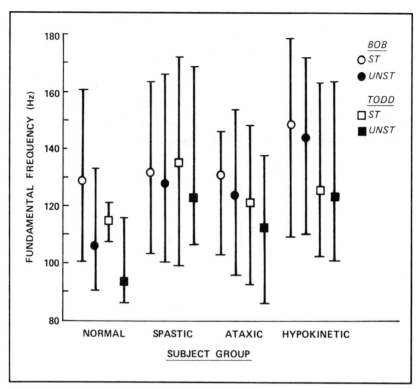

FIGURE 4-2
Means and ranges of the fundamental frequency associated with the vowels in the words *Bob* and *Todd*

Each group was characterized by rather large individual differences for each measure. Figure 4-2 presents an example of the range of measures for the fundamental frequency parameter. While the differences between the stressed and unstressed productions for the normal group are apparent and statistically significant, the differences for the other groups are small by comparison. These differences often failed to reach significance, not unexpectedly, based on the range of values shown in the figure.

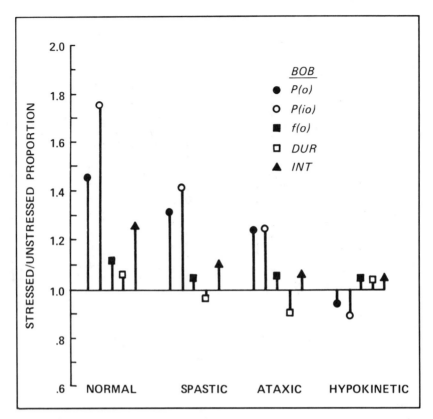

FIGURE 4-3
Ratios of stressed to unstressed mean values for each of five measures for the word *Bob*

In order to compare stressed and unstressed values for the five measures, the stressed-to-unstressed ratios were computed for each measure of the two words. Figure 4-3 shows the ratio for the word *Bob*. A ratio of 1.00 implies equal values for the stressed and unstressed productions. Values larger than 1.00 imply that the stressed condition had the higher value. The figure shows that normal subjects use all five measures to stress the initial word. That is, both the consonant, as measured by the two pressure measures, and the vowel, as measured by fundamental frequency, intensity, and duration, are stressed in the word *Bob*. For the spastic and ataxic subjects, there is evidence of stress on the consonant, but only minimal evidence of stress on the vowel. For the hypokinetic group, the values indicate that they fail to use any of the five parameters to produce stress for the word *Bob*.

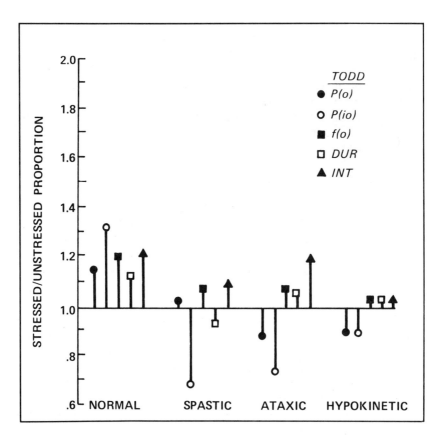

FIGURE 4-4
Ratios of the stressed to unstressed mean values for each of five measures for the word *Todd*

Figure 4-4 shows the ratios of stressed to unstressed values for the word *Todd*. For the normal group, each of the five parameters indicates that the stressed syllable exceeded the unstressed. The ratios for pressure and intensity are smaller in *Todd*, compared to *Bob*; the ratios for fundamental frequency and duration are greater in *Todd*. This may be attributed to the effect of word position within the phrase, or to the effect of voicing on the initial consonant. The fundamental frequency and duration ratios were greater for the unvoiced sample than for the voiced sample.

The spastic and ataxic groups affect final word stress based on the intensity parameter and, to a lesser degree, the fundamental frequency parameter. Unlike their stress patterns for the initial word position, they did not make use of intraoral air pressure or duration to stress a word in the phrase-final position. The hypokinetic group showed essentially no differences in all five parameters studied.

Further examination of the parameters used in the word *Todd* indicates that none of the dysarthric groups had pressure increases in the stressed condition relative to the unstressed. This differs from the initial word in that the spastics and ataxics both used the parameters of articulatory effort to mark stress in the word *Bob*.

DISCUSSION

The results of this study demonstrate that the stress patterns of dysarthric subjects differ from those of normal subjects. The normal subjects of this study used the two consonant- and three vowel-related measures to stress the initial and final words of the three-word phrase. Normal subjects used greater articulatory effort, higher fundamental frequency, longer vowel duration, and greater intensity on the stressed, compared with the unstressed word.

The dysarthric subjects did not use all five prosodic measures to stress initial or final words, and they did not use the same stress patterns for the initial and final words. In some instances, they did not show an increase for a measured parameter in the stressed word when compared with the baseline word. From the findings of all three groups of dysarthric subjects, it is apparent that they are not using the cues for stress that normal subjects use, and the cues which they do invoke are not used to the same degree as they are for the normals.

These data support a model which suggests that dysarthrics use a neuromotor processing system to produce word stress based on compensation rather than enhancement. That is, the normal subjects show an increase in all values for the stressed measures, but all dysarthric groups show a reduction in at least one parameter when they use another parameter(s) to stress a word. More important, these compensatory strategies used by the dysarthrics are not equivocal for each of the three groups.

Based on previous perceptual investigation, the hypokinetic group might be expected to have the most abnormal stress pattern. This group demonstrated only minimal increases in frequency and intensity and they did it at the expense of articulatory effort. Their inability to stress a word using the suprasegmental features associated with normal speech was evident in initial and final positions. This would suggest that previous perceptual characterizations of this group are appropriate (Darley, Aronson, and Brown, 1975). The particular strategy used by these patients in attempting to stress a word requires a reduction in the articulatory effort of consonants when they minimally increase the fundamental frequency, duration or intensity of the vowel.

The spastic and ataxic subjects show a pattern of word stress unlike the hypokinetic group. Again, based on perceptual scaling, these two groups would be expected to utilize at least one of the cues to mark word stress. Their strategy suggests that articulatory effort is used as the primary means to stress the initial word of a phrase. Their modest increases in fundamental frequency and intensity of the stressed words are consistent with perceptual ratings of monopitch and monoloudness. The compromising feature in the initial word for each of these groups is vowel duration. For the final word of a three-word phrase, spastics and ataxics increased fundamental frequency and intensity in the stressed word, but the articulatory effort was compromised and reduced relative to the unstressed word. Thus, these two groups shifted from a consonant-related stress strategy in the initial word of the phrase to a vowel-related strategy for the final word position. This shift is consistent with the general perceptual findings of prosodic insufficiency. The basis for this prosodic insufficiency may have components related to respiratory support, articulatory timing, and utterance length.

The ataxic dysarthrics differed from the spastic group in their use of vowel duration. For the spastics, the vowel duration was reduced in the stressed words compared to baseline. The ataxic group demonstrated a mild tendency to increase duration in the stressed word relative to the baseline in the final word of the phrase; however, just the opposite occurred in the initial word. This group's normal tendency of equalizing duration in all syllables, reported by Kent, Netsell, and Abbs (1979), may account for this finding. In the initial word, this group had relatively large integrated pressure-time measures in the stressed relative to the unstressed word. In the final word, vowel duration increased in the stressed word but integrated pressure-time was less. This finding suggests that groups which equalize one aspect of prosody, namely, duration, use one strategy for phrase initial stress and another for phrase final stress.

The results are encouraging, since they broadly reflect perceptual observations previously reported. Despite the high variability in each group, these methods and measures described offer an approach to the quantification of dysarthric speech.

In summary, the stress patterns of spastic, ataxic, and hypokinetic dysarthric subjects differ from normal subjects. Normal speakers use consonant- and vowel-based prosodic cues to mark stress in initial and final words of a phrase. Hypokinetic subjects show almost no ability to use either type of cue to stress words. Spastic and ataxic dysarthrics use a complex strategy based on compensatory behaviors. When they use consonant-related cues to stress a word, vowel-related cues are reduced relative to a baseline condition. This occurs in the initial word position. For the final word position, the two groups switch to a vowel-based stress code, resulting in reduced consonant articulatory effort. The use of vowel duration to impart word stress differentiates the spastic from the ataxic subject. Finally, this investigation is consistent with the perceptual analyses of these groups previously reported.

GLOSSARY

Stress — An abstract entity generated by phonological rules indicating the relative importance of different syllables and usually reflected by a greater degree of articulatory effort. Synonymous with stress in spoken language are emphasis, prominence, importance, and significance.

Intraoral air pressure — the build-up of air pressure in the oral cavity behind the place of consonant articulation.

Integrated pressure-time — The measure of intraoral air pressure when integrated over the entire utterance from rise above baseline through the peak and return to baseline. The value is measured in units of pressure per units of time; e.g. Cm H2O/sec.

REFERENCES

Barnes, G. Suprasegmental and prosodic considerations in motor speech. In W. Berry (Ed.), *Clinical dysarthria*, San Diego, College-Hill Press, 1983.

Brown, W., & McGlone, R. Aerodynamic and acoustic study of stress in sentence production. *Journal of the Acoustical Society of America,* 1974, *56,* 971-974.

Brown, W., & Shearer, W. Constancy of intraoral air pressure related to integrated pressure-time measures. *Folia Phoniatrica,* 1970, *22,* 49-57.

Darley, F., Aronson, A., & Brown, J. *Motor speech disorders.* Philadelphia: Saunders, 1975.

Fry, D. Duration and intensity as physical correlates of linguistic stress. *Journal of the Acoustical Society of America*, 1955, *27*, 765-768.

Kent, R., Netsell, R., & Abbs, J. Acoustic characteristics of dysarthria associated with cerebellar disease. *Journal of Speech and Hearing Research*, 1979, *22*, 627-648.

Liebermann, P. *Intonation, perception and language.* Cambridge: MIT Press, 1967.

Muller, E., & Brown, W. Variations in the supraglottal air pressure waveform and their articulatory interpretation. *SMCL Reprint,* University of Wisconsin, 1980.

Murry, R., & Brown, W. Peak intraoral air pressure in whispered stop consonants. *Journal of Phonetics*, 1976, *4*, 183-187.

Rabiner, L., Levitt, H., & Rosenberg, A. Investigation of stress patterns for speech synthesis by rule. *Journal of the Acoustical Society of America*, 1969, *45*, 92-101.

Yorkston, K., Beukelman, D., & Minifie, F. Computer analysis of some acoustic parameters of dysarthric speech. Paper presented at the convention of the American Speech-Language-Hearing Association, Atlanta, November 1979.

ACKNOWLEDGEMENT

This study was supported by the Veteran's Administration. The author wishes to thank Michael Caligiuri for his assistance in this research.

5

The Frequency of Verbal and Acoustic Adjustments Used by Cerebral Palsied Dysarthric Adults When Faced with Communicative Failure

Beth M. Ansel
Malcolm R. McNeil
Chauncey J. Hunker
Diane M. Bless

INTRODUCTION

Within the confines of our speech and language system, there is a range of intelligibility that is acceptable. Those individuals on the margins and those who fall outside this range may not only experience the failure of the communicative act, but may experience rejection, anxiety, frustration, and may even withdraw from communicative interactions (Gilmore, 1974). Decreased intelligibility is a common result of several communicative disorders associated with neurogenic and structural anomalies. It occurs in a substantial number of adults, and has been suggested by some to be the rudimentary and paramount target for treatment (Rosenbek and LaPointe, 1978).

The dysarthrias may be among the most severe disorders in their effect on intelligibility because of the diverse clinical features which are manifestations of impairments across several components of the speech production system. Tikofsky and Tikofsky (1964) compared intelligibility scores of normal and dysarthric speakers and found significant differences between the two groups. Their results indicated that the motor speech disorders significantly impair the transmission of speech such that normal listeners cannot readily adapt to the unfamiliar articulatory and phonatory patterns of the speakers, nor can they benefit much from practice.

Several studies have systematically investigated the factors influencing estimates of dysarthric speech intelligibility and their effect on functional communication. Results have shown that listener experience, word predictability, utterance length, and listener familiarity with the speech sample are all contextual factors that serve to influence the intelligibility estimates for disorderd speakers (Duffy and Giolas, 1974; Platt, Andrews, Young, and Neilson, 1978; Platt, Andrew, Young, and Quinn, 1980; Beukelman and Yorkston, 1979, and 1980; Rentchler and Mann, 1980.

Beukelman and Yorkston (1979, 1980) conducted a series of studies directed towards examining the relationship between information transfer and speech intelligibility as measured by single-word and paragraph transcription across a wide severity range of dysarthric speakers. They found a close relationship between intelligibility and information transfer, which they felt supported the use of intelligibility scores as a functional index of communicative performance. Further, Yorkston and Beukelman (1978) found that although connected speech had been observed to be easier to understand by several authors (Duffy and Giolas, 1974; Miller, Heise, and Lichten, 1950), this did not hold across the entire severity range. They reported that

> there is an interaction between dysarthria severity and intelligibility on sentences versus words, i.e., the most intelligible speakers tended to score higher on sentence transcription rather than single word transcription and the least intelligible speakers received higher scores on single words (Yorkston and Beukelman, 1978; p. 510).

They offered the explanation that relatively intelligible speakers are aided by context and that connected speech may provide listeners with enough redundant information to allow them to predict a word in context more accurately than a word in isolation. Thus, the length and completeness of an utterance may be an important consideration in successful communication. The phonemic and linguistic cues and redundancy carried in the complete message may better enable the listener to recognize individual sounds or words in the message that are difficult to understand, or to fill in where the message is unintelligible. This supposition is in accordance with that of Platt et al. (1978). On the other hand, for the more unintelligible speaker, a short phrase or single word may facilitate the listeners' ability to process the phonemic cues at a less complex level.

Rehabilitation programs designed to improve the oral communication skills of these populations have generally focused directly on articulatory and prosodic parameters of speech production. Descriptions of therapy programs rarely include suggestions for working directly on the speaker's ability to modify contextual aspects of an utterance to adapt to the needs of the listener. The reason contextual aspects are not considered an integral part of therapy is not clear. Clinicians may assume that, since children are able to adapt to the needs of the listener, communicatively handicapped adults should be able to make similar modifications without specific training (Gallagher, 1977; Garvey, 1975). In addition, clinicians may assume that, since treatment incorporates such parameters as pitch, loudness, and phonetic placement, the speech-impaired individual learns automatically to work to maximum production capacity and has no need to monitor those language-based modifications that have been found to assist the listener in understanding (e.g., listener experience, word familiarity, utterance, length, etc.). Both of these assumptions may be false.

Failure to incorporate contextual factors influencing speech intelligibility as it relates both to the listener and to the structure and function of language may present several problems. First, it may yield an unrealistic assessment of functional communication by clinicians. The studies reviewed concerning naive and sophisticated listeners (Beukelman and Yorkston, 1980; Platt et al., 1980), as well as those dealing with passage familiarity (Beukelman and Yorkston, 1980), indicate that the clinician's perception may not be the best guide in judging functional communication. Moreover, if dysarthric speakers are not aware of those factors believed to facilitate communicative effectiveness with listeners, they may have an unrealistic expectation of their effectiveness in dealing with naive listeners.

Secondly, the importance of contextual factors which serve to increase intelligibility, such as word predictability, listener experience, listener familiarity with the speech sample, and utterance length (Duffy and Giolas, 1974; Beukelman and Yorkston, 1979, 1980; Yorkston and Beukelman, 1978; Platt et al., 1978 and 1980), are seemingly ignored.

Third, without this perspective, therapeutic procedures appropriate to different degrees of severity are not likely to be utilized; for example, use of complete sentences to increase intelligibility of mildly impaired, or the use of short words and phrases for severely impaired (Yorkston and Beukelman, 1978; Beukelman and Yorkston, 1980.

While speech/language pathologists have recognized the ability of normally developing children to adapt to the needs of the listener and produce messages that can be understood and responded to, no such verbal adjustments have been investigated for children and adults with motor speech disorders. To our knowledge, no studies have addressed spontaneous contextual adaptations to the intelligibility problem, the effect of these adaptations on functional communication, or whether these adapations can be learned.

As an initial step in examining contextual adaptations, this study was designed to determine if and how adult speakers with reduced speech intelligibility adapted to communication failure. This was accomplished by quantifying the verbal and intensity adjustments employed by the subjects in response to communicative failures. Additionally, this study sought to determine the relationships between the frequency with which a particular verbal adjustment and query type were employed, and the relationship between verbal adjustment and the severity of the intelligibility impairment.

METHODS

Ten congenitally dysarthric cerebral-palsied adult speakers, who were athetoid, spastic, and mixed types, served as subjects. These subjects were selected to reflect a range of severity in terms of speech intelligibility. Only subjects who used verbal speech as their sole method of communication were included. Subjects' ages ranged from 20 years to 47 years with a mean age of 29.4. The level of speech intelligibility was quantified by having the subjects read five sentences randomly generated from a grid developed for a home practice program by Yorkston and Beukelman (1981). The utterances were recorded and subsequently transcribed by ten listeners unfamiliar with the type of speaker and the stimulus materials. Intelligibility was an objective measure of the percentage of words correctly transcribed orthographically. The mean score of the five sentences from each listener was calculated to yield an overall intelligibility score for each subject. The intelligibility ratings along with biographical and selected physiological data are summarized in Table 5-1. For descriptive purposes each speaker was given an assessment battery consisting of language, cognitive, and articulatory tasks, as well as estimates of subglottal pressure and intensity ranges to help eliminate alternative explanations of the derived data (Table 5-2). The descriptive battery is summarized in Appendix A.

TABLE 5-1

Age, sex, formal education, dysarthria type, intelligibility rating, subglottal pressure, and sound pressure level ranges for ten experimental subjects

Subject	Age (yrs.)	Sex	Formal Education (yrs.)	Dysarthria Type	Intelligibility Rating	Subglottal Pressure	SPL Range (dB)
1	47	M	12	Spastic, Athetoid	63%	10cm H_2O / 6 seconds	55-90
2	37	M	16	Spastic	88%	8cm H_2O / 6 seconds	55-90
3	34	M	12	Spastic	43%	10cm H_2O / 8 seconds	55-98
4	31	M	20	Spastic, Athetoid	85%	7cm H_2O / 7 seconds	55-85
5	28	M	12	Spastic	93%	10cm H_2O / 10 seconds	55-85
6	26	M	13	Spastic	17%	7cm H_2O / 6 seconds	60-94
7	25	F	12	Spastic, Athetoid	44%	7cm H_2O / 6 seconds	55-85
8	25	F	16	Spastic, Athetoid	90%	8cm H_2O / 7 seconds	50-90
9	21	M	12	Athetoid	42%	7cm H_2O / 8 seconds	60-105
10	20	F	13	Athetoid	62%	6cm H_2O / 5 seconds	55-95

TABLE 5-2
Summary of results of the Ravens Coloured Matrices Test, Word Fluency Measure, Detroit Test of Learning Aptitude Subtest 19, Goldman-Fristoe Test of Articulation, Shortened Porch Index of Communicative Ability, Content Units Per Minutes, and the Ammons Full-Range Picture Vocabulary Test for ten experimental subjects

Subject	Ravens (% correct)	Word Fluency Measure (total)	Detroit (% correct)	Goldman-Fristoe (% correct)	SPICA (O.A.X)	Content Units (per minute)	Ammons (% 'tile)
1	83	45	91	65	11.60	15	80th
2	64	34	80	97	12.89	13	80th
3	33	32	59	80	11.52	17	22nd
4	97	91	100	80	13.98	14	100th
5	81	32	60	74	12.55	14	25th
6	89	43	85	07	7.28	15	78th
7	33	18	60	28	8.62	14	1st
8	83	73	89	95	13.63	20	90th
9	81	41	70	61	12.62	16	22nd
10	92	51	90	76	12.17	17	90th

Twelve times during a 25-minute audio-recorded conversational interview, the experimenter indiciated an inability to understand what the speaker had said, and asked "What ?" "Excuse Me ?" or "I'm sorry?". Of the 12 queries, 9 were single indications of communicative failures, and 3 were multiple requests (three consecutive) indicating further clarification was still required. Each query response was compared to the original utterance to determine the verbal adjustments made by the subjects to accommodate the listener. The verbal adjustments were examined and classified into one of 31 categories. These categories included 10 basic ones, with 21 additional categories resulting from simultaneous employment of two or more verbal adjustments. The following were the ten basic categories as operationally defined for this investigation:

1. **Total Repetition** - entire utterance is reiterated verbatim.

2. **Partial Repetition/Word** - one word of the utterance is reiterated.

3. **Partial Repetition/Phrase** - a segment of the utterance is reiterated in the same words.

4. **Elaboration** - utterance is expressed with greater complexity, fullness of detail. More syllable units are utilized. Not merely a restatement.

5. **Spelling of Word** - naming of letters of the word in order.

6. **Convergent Phrase** - use of a phrase wherein information is preserved with change to fewer number of syllable units (e.g., "This guy and I both" changed to "We both").

7. **Synonym and Word Convergence** - use of a single word of the same language that has nearly the same meaning in some or all senses, a semantic change.

8. **Syntactic Revision** - utterance differs structurally from the form of the original utterance, i.e., word reordering, change from passive to active, change from negative to affirmative.

9. **Simplification** - abbreviation of a word or phrase e.g., *classroom* is changed to *room*, *occupational therapist* is changed to *O.T.*

10. **Semantic Specification** - utterance is expressed with greater complexity, fullness of detail with fewer number of syllable units, e.g., "We talk about our problems"is changed to "It's a support group."

All 31 verbal adjustments categories are listed in Table 5-3.

TABLE 5-3
Thirty-one verbal adjustment categories

Verbal Adjustment

1.   Total Repetition
2.   Partial Repetition/Word
3.   Partial Repetition/Phrase
4.   Synonym and Word Convergence
5.   Convergent Phrase
6.   Elaboration
7.   Semantic Specification
8.   Syntactic Revision
9.   Spelling
10. Simplification
11. Synonym and Word Convergence and Elaboration
12. Partial Repetition/Phrase and Elaboration
13. Partial Repetition/Phrase and Syntactic Revision
14. Partial Repetition/Phrase and Convergent Phrase
15. Partial Repetition/Phrase and Synonym and Word Convergence
16. Partial Repetition/Phrase and Semantic Specification
17. Partial Repetition/Word and Elaboration
18. Partial Repetition/Word and Semantic Specification
19. Partial Repetition/Word and Synonym and Word Convergence
20. Partial Repetition/Word and Convergenct Phrase
21. Partial Repetition/Word and Spelling
22. Total Repetition and Elaboration
23. Elaboration and Syntactic Revision
24. Synonym and Word Convergence and Syntactic Revision
25. Partial Repetition/Phrase and Elaboration and Simplification
26. Partial Repetition/Phrase and Synonym and Word Convergence and Elaboration

27. Partial Repetition/ Phrase and Convergent Phrase and Elaboration
28. Partial Repetition/ Phrase and Elaboration and Syntactic Revision
29. Partial Repetition/ Phrase and Elaboration and Spelling
30. Partial Repetition/ Phrase and Synonym and Word Convergence and Syntactic Revision
31. Partial Repetition/ Phrase and Synonym and Word Convergence and Simplification

In addition to the verbal adjustments, the intensity of each utterance was analyzed to determine if that parameter was manipulated in response to ineffective communication interactions. The pre-query and post-query utterances were digitized, and the overall intensity levels were calculated via the Vocal. Manipulation Program for Utterance Tape Production (cf. Ansel, 1981), and compared within and across subjects and query tapes.

RESULTS

Response Categories

From each subject, 9 responses were obtained from both single and multiple queries, totaling 18 individual utterances. Each of the subjects' 18 responses were subsequently analyzed and classified into one of the 31 verbal adjustment categories. This classification provided frequency data for each verbal adjustment with respect to query type. These data were submitted to a two-factor analysis of variance (Marascuilo, 1971) of query type and verbal adjustments. These ANOVA results are presented in Table 5-4.

TABLE 5-4

Analysis of variance of query type and verbal adjustment categories

Source of Variation	Degree of Freedom	Sums of Squares	Mean Squares	F
Query Type (QT)	1	0.002	0.002	.007
Verbal Adjustment Category (VAC)	30	145.671	4.856	18.394
QT x VAC	30	8.548	0.285	.001
Error	558	147.100	0.264	
Total	619	301.321		

Query Type—The main effect of query type (F=.007, 1.558; p > 0.05) was not significant, indicating that response variability was not due to single or multiple queries.

Verbal Adjustments—The main effect of verbal adjustments (F= 18.394, 30,558; p < 0.05) was significant, indicating that the variability in responses was due to the use of a variety of linguistic forms and adjustments. Post hoc analysis between verbal adjustment categories comparisons were performed using the least-significant-differences method for multi-factorial comparisons (Marscuilo, 1971). The following results were obtained at significance level of p=0.05: a) the production of categbry 3, Partial Repetition of a Phrase, and category 1, Total Repetition, were significantly different from the remaining verbal categories; b) the production of category 12, Partial Repetition of a Phrase with Elaboration, was not significantly different from categories 2, Partial Repetition of a Word, and 22, Total Repetition with Elaboration, but was significantly different from the remaining verbal adjustment categories; c) the frequency of occurrence of the remaining 27 verbal categories was not significantly different from one another. Figure 5-1 displays the relative frequency of the categorized verbal adjustment productions. This descriptive summary illustrates that the verbal adjustment represented by

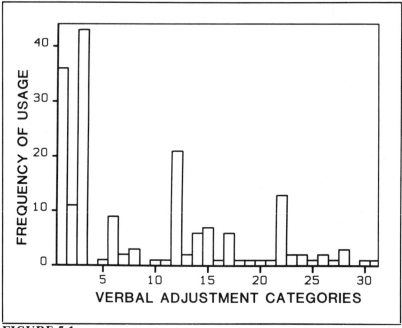

FIGURE 5-1
Histogram of frequency of verbal adjustments utilized

category 3 was most frequently used (24%), followed by categories 1 (20%), 12 (12%), 22 (7%), and 2 (6%), respectively. The remaining verbal adjustments categories were each used less than 5%.

Verbal Adjustments/Query Type — There was no statistically significant evidence that these two factors, verbal adjustments and query type, interacted (F=1.08, 30, 558; p > 0.05). That is, the particular verbal response did not vary as a function of query type. Further qualitative analysis of the verbal adjustments used following successive communicative failures did not reveal any specific sequential pattern of verbal adjusments in the responses.

Verbal Adjustment/Subject Intelligibility

Intelligibility scores from sentence transcriptions were computed for each subject, and are presented in Table 5-1. As shown, subject intelligibility scores ranged from 17% to 93% (mean % words correctly transcribed). These differences in intelligibility ratings reflected the wide range of the severity of subjects. Intelligibility scores were correlated with the frequency with which identified verbal adjustment categories were utilized. As shown in Appendix B, correlations were repeated for each of the 31 verbal adjustment categories. All correlations were very low and non-significant at the 0.05 level. Even the two highest correlation accounted for only 33% and 35% of the explained variance. This suggests that there was little relationship between the type of verbal response utilized and the overall intelligibility of each subject's speech.

Intensity Adjustments

The intensity level was calculated for each utterance made prior to a query and for each utterance immediately following the query. The utterances were identified as pre- and post-query responses, respectively. These data were grouped into pre- and post-query responses at the single query level, and pre- and post-query responses at the multiple query level. Each of these sets of data were submitted to a two-factor analysis of variance. Results are presented in Tables 5-5 and 5-6, respectively.

TABLE 5-5
Analysis of variance of pre- and post-query responses and subjects for single query situations

Source of Variation	Degree of Freedom	Sums of Squares	Mean Squares	F
Pre- and Post-Query Response	1	36.5	36.5	3.02
Subjects	9	6442.4	715.8	89.50*
Pand PQR x Subjects	9	122.5	13.6	1.12
Error	160	1931.6	12.1	
Total	179	8532.9		

*Significant p ≤ .05

TABLE 5-6
Analysis of variance of pre- and post-query responses and subjects for multiple query situations

Source of Variation	Degree of Freedom	Sums of Squares	Mean Squares	F
Pre- and Post-Query Response	3	11.5	3.8	.215
Subjects	9	2912.7	323.6	18.280*
Pand PQR x Subjects	27	175.1	6.5	.370
Error	80	1412.0	17.7	
Total	119	4511.3		

*Significant p ≤ .05

Pre- and Post-Query Intensity Level — The overall average intensity of the single pre-query responses was 51 dB, and 52 dB for the overall average intensity single post-query responses. Pre- and post- multiple query intensity means were 52 dB and 53 dB, respectively. As summarized in Tables 5-5 and 5-6, the ANOVA results for these pre- and post-, single and multiple query intensity levels were not significant [single: ($F=3.02$, 1, 160; $p > 0.05$) and multiple: ($F=0.215$, 3, 80; $p > 0.05$)], suggesting that the intensity levels used by these subjects did not vary systematically as a function of pre-versus post- or single versus multiple query types imposed upon them.

Intensity Level Among Subjects — The mean overall average intensity of the single query responses for all subjects combined was 51 dB, and 52 dB for the mean overall average intensity of the multiple query responses for all subjects combined. The mean overall average intensity ranges were 39 dB to 58 dB and 40 dB to 57 dB for the single and multiple queries, respectively. ANOVA results among subjects were significant in single ($F=89.5$, 9, 160; $p < 0.05$) and also multiple ($F=18.28$, 9, 8; $p > 0.05$) query situations, indicating that the significance was attributed to the overall intensity level differences between individual subjects, and not differences within subjects on either query type.

Pre- and Post-Query Intensity Level/Subject — There was no statistically significant evidence to support the notion that pre- and post- query intensity level interacted for either the single query ($F=1.12$, 9, 160; $p > 0.05$), or the multiple query ($F=0.37$, 27, 80; $p > 0.05$) situations. This indicated that the pre- and post-query intensity level for each individual subject did not vary systematically, but, that the pre- and post-query intensity levels among subjects did vary systematically. For example, for subject 1, the overall average intensity of the single pre-query responses was 39 dB, and the overall average intensity of the single post-query responses was also 39 dB. For subject 8, the overall average intensity of the single pre-query responses was 58 dB, and the overall average intensity of the single post-query responses was also 58 dB. These findings illustrate that although there was no significant difference in the pre- and post-query intensity level within subjects, there were, however, significant differences among subjects.

Intensity Adjustments/Speaker Intellgibility

It was found that the average intensity levels were not significantly different prior to or following the query, for either the single or multiple query situations. This held true across all 10 subjects. Therefore, there was no need to correlate speaker intelligibility with intensity adjustments.

Direction of Intensity Adjustments

A two-tail sign test (Marascuilo, 1971) was used to compare the adjustment of intensity in the positive direction with the adjustment of intensity in the negative direction. Prior to employing the sign test, independence between pre- and post-query responses was established with the use of x-y scatter plots. Comparisons were made across subjects as well as within subjects. Comparisons also included responses to single queries, multiple queries, and the two different query types combined. Results of each comparison were not significant at the = 0.05 level, indicating that the direction of intensity adjustments was not systematically utilized in response to either query types.

Additionally, a two-tailed sign test was used to compare the direction of intensity adjustments that had occurred with category 1, Total Repetition, alone. Results of this sign test were not significant at the = 0.05 level, yielding further evidence that directional intensity adjustments were not systematically utilized.

Reliability

For the verbal adjustment categorization of all responses for all 10 subjects, intra-judge reliability of categorizing verbal adjustments was checked on three occasions, each separated by a time period of two weeks. Agreement of 100% between categorizations was reached. Inter-judge agreement of 99% on the same measure was also achieved for two judges. A graduate student in Speech Pathology, who had been trained with a verbal and written description of the verbal adjustment categories, served as one judge. The first author served as the second judge.

The entire Short Version of the Porch Index of Communicative Ability (SPICA) was scored a second time on one subject, separated by a time period of one week. The resultant difference of 0.06 between the two overall average scores was considered to be reliable.

One naive listener rescored the subject's speech intelligibility from the master sentence tape two weeks after the first scoring procedure. Agreement of 98% between the two different scoring procedures was reached.

DISCUSSION

Our findings have shown that: (1) the verbal adjustments employed were not dependent upon single or multiple query types; (2) four verbal adjustments were utilized substantively more frequently than others, namely, total repetition, partial repetition of a phrase, partial repetition of a phrase with elaboration, and total repetition with elaboration, which accounted for 63% of all categories used; (3) the selection of verbal adjustments did not vary as a function of speaker intelligibility; and (4) the adjustments of intensity were not systematically utilized.

The speakers in our study did not differentially alter their verbal or acoustic behavior when faced with either single or consecutive instances of communicative failure. The reason for this is not readily apparent. It may be that these speakers had not identified types of response adjustments that are most consistently effective for them. Or, as the literature suggests, that because intelligibility is so dependent upon listener experience and word predictability, it is virtually impossible for these speech intelligibility-impaired individuals to predict modifications that will be most effective for them in different situations. Alternatively, it may be a result of the speakers' perception of their own intelligibility. In support of this notion is the observation that when questioned regarding the amount of difficulty they perceived their listeners to have in understanding their speech, each subject responded that the listener had little difficulty. Subjects, regardless of their rating on the formal articulation test or by naive listener estimates of intelligibility, responded similarly.

With a continuing breakdown in communication, there was no sequential pattern of adjustments that these speakers used in their attempts to be understood. A possible explanation may be that since these speakers constantly function at a reduced intelligibility level, being faced with communicative failure is not an unusual occurrence for them. One may speculate that through the course of their lifetimes, they have become accustomed, and, possibly, desensitized to indices of communication breakdown. Because of this desensitization to repeated questioning, they may handle each request for information on an utterance-by-utterance basis, viewing a multiple query situation as merely a sequence of isolated single queries.

Other possible factors in explaining why the linguistic adjustments employed were not dependent upon single or multiple query type, may be each subject's perception of the cause of the impaired intelligibility during this particular interaction. It is usual during the course of a conversational interaction for the listener to alert the speaker when communication failure has taken place, through the use of facial or body gestures or direct questioning. All subjects were queried after they had completed their utterance. The queries were purposefully non-directive and, therefore, gave the speakers no specific cues as to where the difficulty was. Because of the benign nature of the query, one might speculate that these speakers did not know, in the multiple query situations, if the query was in response to their previous utterance or to the earlier utterance that triggered the succession of multiple queries. These results would again indicate that the speakers in this study handled each response independent of any prior response. In view of the independent relationship between the pre- and post-query responses, one could conclude that these speakers viewed the multiple queries not as a succession of related queries, but as isolated queries following one another.

Conversational Interaction Responsibilities

Our results indicate that impaired speakers may need more specific information to shape their further responses. This suggests that speakers as well as listeners have responsibilities within conversational interactions. For truly effective communication, the speaker—especially the speech intelligibility-impaired speaker—must educate the listener, and alert him/her to indicate specifically what is not understood and where the communication breakdown has taken place.

Several authors (Yorkston and Beukelman, 1978; Platt et al., 1978) have shown that the most intelligible dysarthric speakers tended to score higher on sentence production rather than single word production, and the least intelligible speakers received higher scores on single words. Thus, the length and completeness of an utterance may be an important consideration in successful communication. These authors offer the explanation that for the most intelligible speaker, the phonemic and linguistic cues and redundancy carried in the complete message may better enable the listener to recognize individual sounds or words in the message that are difficult to understand, or to fill in where the message is intelligible. On the other hand, for the more unintelligible speaker, a short phrase or single word may facilitate the listener's ability to process the phonemic cues at a less complex level.

While the dysarthric speakers in this study altered their verbal responses to queries, they did not modify the linguistic structure of their responses in the manner predicted from previous studies. Of the four verbal adjustments that were utilized most frequently, elaborative adjustments were used as commonly as succinct adjustments, i.e., partial repetition of a word, and total repetition with elaboration. These four categories comprised 63% of the total responses, of that 44% remained the same or reduced in length, and 19% were longer in word content. These length adjustments of the verbal utterances, however, did not vary as a function of speaker intelligibility, as would be expected. The dysarthric speakers in this study did not incorporate the utterance modifications that the literature suggests would be most effective for them. Thus, it appears that this is a more complex issue than is generally realized. The findings of this study would indicate that linguistic context is also of importance, and that the function which language serves must be considered.

Intensity Analysis

Intuitively, one may predict that when faced with communicative failure, as evidenced by a query, speakers might adjust the intensity level of their responses, especially when repeating the total message. This was not found with this subject population. Netsell and Hixon (1978, p.329) observed that "individuals who can generate and sustain 5 cm of H_2O for 5 seconds with a leak tube have sufficient pressure capabilities to meet speech requirements." Based upon sub-glottal air pressure estimates and sound pressure level ranges, it is reasonable to expect that the subjects in this study were physiologically able to make adjustments of intensity. One reason they did not might be that these subjects had not found adjustments of intensity to be of use to them in responses to queries. Perhaps when faced with communicative failure, these speakers perceived that it was, in fact, the message content and not the intensity parameter that was interfering with the information transfer. Therefore, they adjusted the verbal content rather than the intensity level.

Rosenbek and LaPointe (1978) view the goal of treatment for dysarthric speakers to be compensated intelligibility. Rehabilitation programs designed to improve the oral communication skills of these populations have generally focused directly on perceptual and physiological parameters of speech production. While this is certainly the essential focus of treatment, intelligibility obviously encompasses more than just the physiological components of speech. Although the dysarthrias are motor speech problems and not language disorders, the present study suggests that one must also consider language components in their treatment. It may be that clinicians need to incorporate the speaker's ability to modify linguistic aspects of an utterance to adapt to the need of the listener — a pragmatic component of speech intelligibility.

This study was an initial step towards investigating verbal adjustments and adjustments of intensity used by dysarthric individuals during instances of communicative failure. The innovative classification system used in this investigation might be expected to have equally useful application to other populations with speech intelligibility impairment. As yet, it is not certain to what extent these verbal and intensity adjustments actually functioned as compensatory behaviors to increase speech intelligibility quantitatively. Such conclusions must await more detailed analysis of the present data, which is currently in progress.

REFERENCES

Ammons, R., & Ammons, H. *Full-range picture vocabulary test.* Missoula, MT: Psychological Test Specialists, 1948.

Ansel, B. Frequency of verbal and acoustic adjustments used by cerebral-palsied-dysarthric adults when faced with communicative failure. Unpublished master's thesis, University of Wisconsin-Madison, 1981.

Baker, H., & Leland, B. *Detroit tests of learning aptitude.* Indianapolis: The Bobbs-Merrill Company, Inc., 1977.

Beukelman, D., & Yorkston, K. The relationship between information transfer and speech intelligibility of dysarthric speakers. *Journal of Communication Disorders,* 1979, *12,* 189-196.

Beukelman, D., & Yorkston, K. The influence of passage familiarity on intelligibility estimates of dysarthric speech. *Journal of Communication Disorders,* 1980, *13,* 33-41.

DiSimoni, F., Keith, R., & Darley, F. Prediction of PICA overall score by short version of the test. *Journal of Speech and Hearing Research,* 1980, *23,* 511-516.

Duffy, J., & Giolas, T. Sentence intelligibility as a function of key word selection. *Journal of Speech and Hearing Research,* 1974, *17,* 631-637.

Gallagher, T. Revision behaviors in the speech of normal children developing language. *Journal of Speech and Hearing Research,* 1977, *20,* 303-318.

Garvey, C. The contingent query: A dependent act in conversation. In M. Lewis & L. Rosenblum (Eds.), *Interaction, conversation and the development of language.* New York: John Wiley and Sons, 1975.

Gilmore, S. Social and vocational acceptability of esophageal speakers compared to normal speakers. *Journal of Speech and Hearing Research,* 1974, *17,* 599-607.

Goldman, R., & Fristoe, M. *Goldman-Fristoe test of articulation.* American Guidance Service, Inc., 1972.

Goodglass, H., & Kaplan, E. *Boston diagnostic aphasia examination.* Philadelphia: Lee and Febiger, 1972.

Marascuilo, L.A. *Statistical methods for behavioral science research.* New York: McGraw-Hill Inc., 1971.

Miller, G., Heise, G., & Lichten, W. The intelligibility of speech as a function of the test material. *Journal of Experimental Psychology*, 1950, *41*, 329-335.

Netsell, R., & Hixon, T. A noninvasive method for clinically estimating subglottal air pressure. *Journal of Speech and Hearing Disorders*, 1978, *43*, 326-330.

Platt, L., Andrews, G., Young, M., & Neilson, P. The measurement of speech impairment of adults with cerebral palsy. *Folia Phoniatrica.* 1978, *30*, 50-58.

Platt, L., Andrews, G., Young, M., & Quinn, P. Dysarthria of adult cerebral palsy: 1. Intelligibility and articulatory impairment. *Journal of Speech and Hearing Research*, 1980, *23*, 28-40.

Ravens, J. *Coloured progressive matrices.* London: H.K. Lewis, 1962.

Rentschler, G., & Mann, M. The effect of glossectomy on intelligibility of speech and oral perception. *Journal of Oral Surgery*, 1980, *38*, 344-353.

Rosenbek, J., & LaPointe, L. The dysarthrias: Description, diagnosis and treatment. In D. Johns (Ed.), *Clinical management of neurogenic communication disorders.* Boston: Little, Brown and Company, 1978.

Tikofsky, R., & Tikofsky R. Intelligibility measures of dysarthric speech, *Journal of Speech and Hearing Research*, 1964, *7*, 325-333.

Wertz, R., Keith, R., & Custer, D. *Word fluency measure (2nd Version).* Unpublished. Rochester, MN: Mayo Clinic.

Yorkston, K., & Beukelman, D. A comparison of techniques for measuring intelligibility of dysarthric speech. *Journal of Communication Disorder*, 1978, *11*, 499-512.

Yorkston, K., & Beukelman, D. An analysis of connected speech samples of aphasic and normal speakers. *Journal of Speech and Hearing Disorders*, 1980, *45*, 27-36.

Yorkston, K., & Beukelman, D. Ataxic dysarthria: Treatment sequences based on ntelligibility and prosodic considerations. *Journal of Speech and Hearing Disorders*, 1981, *46*, 398-404.

ACKNOWLEDGEMENT

This work was supported in part by the National Institute of Health Grant NS-13274-05.

APPENDIX A

The descriptive battery consisted of the following formal tests:

1. The Ravens Coloured Progressive Matrices Test (Raven, 1962) assessed nonverbal reasoning.

2. The Goldman-Fristoe Test of Articulation (Goldman and Fristoe, 1972) allowed for further description of each subject's articulatory ability.

3. The Ammons Full-Range Picture Vocabulary Test Form A (Ammons and Ammons, 1948) was used as a vehicle for estimating receptive vocabulary.

4. The Detroit Tests of Learning Aptitude Subtest Nineteen (Baker and Leland, 1967) was used to estimate each subject's ability to use synonyms so as to further document their knowledge of linguistics which might potentially be used as a linguistic device when faced with communicative failure.

5. The Short Version of the Porch Index Communicative Ability (SPICA), Second Version (DiSimoni, Keith, and Darley, 1980) assessed language performance and ability to perform across modalities. SPICA was administered in a slightly modified form to accommodate some of the motor deficits of the subjects, and was scored by a trained and reliable scorer. On the SPICA, all subject's responses were characterized by scores of 4, 7, and 14. Specifically, over the 10 subjects, 26% to 74% of the overall scores were 4, 7, or 14. Two subjects were motorically unable to attempt any of the graphic tests. These types of scores are indicative of motoric disturbances rather than cognitive abilities and, therefore, contributed to the depressed scores of the severe motorically involved subjects.

6. Word Fluency Measures (Wertz, Keith and Custer, 1971) was used to further establish the subjects' knowledge and use of word association and retrieval.

7. One minute speech samples were elicited through a picture description task Cookie Thief picture, Boston Diagnostic Aphasia Examination) and analyzed (Yorkston and Beukelman, 1980) to quantify the amount of information conveyed via the total number of content units contained in the picture description sample.

8. The average of three repetitions of speech, just above a whisper to measure sound pressure level for minimal vocal intensity control, and the average of three repetitions of "Hey, you" shouted as loudly as possible to measure the sound pressure level for maximum vocal intensity control.

9. Estimates of subglottal air pressure were obtained by using a U-tube manometer with a leak tube held in one side of the mouth. The subjects were instructed to blow into both tubes, keeping the lips tightly sealed around the tubes, and maintain prescribed pressure level 5 cm H_2O for the specified duration of 5 seconds (Netsell and Hixon, 1978).

The order of the task presentation was randomized to prevent any order effect.

APPENDIX B

Correlations for each of the 31 verbal adjustment categories for 10 experimental subjects

Verbal Adjustment	r	R2
1.Total Repetition	0.152	0.023
2.Partial Repetition/Word	0.131	0.017
3.Partial Repetition/Phrase	0.195	0.038
4.Synonym and Word Convergence	---	---
5.Convergent Phrase	0.009	0.000
6.Elaboration	0.576	0.332
7.Semantic Specification	0.004	0.000
8.Syntactic Revision	0.256	0.066
9.Spelling	---	---
10.Simplification	0.343	0.118
11.Synonym and Word Convergence and Elaboration	0.280	0.078
12.Partial Repetition/Phrase and Elaboration	0.156	0.243

13. Partial Repetition/Phrase and
    Syntactic Revision   0.301   0.091
14. Partial Repetition/Phrase and
    Convergent Phrase   0.244   0.060
15. Partial Repetition/Phrase and
    Synonym and Word Convergence   0.118   0.014
16. Partial Repetition/Phrase and
    Semantic Specification   0.343   0.118
17. Partial Repetition/Word and
    Elaboration   0.387   0.150
18. Partial Repetition/Word and Semantic
    Specification   0.370   0.137
19. Partial Repetition/Word and Synonym
    and Word Convergence   0.619   0.383
20. Partial Repetition/Word and
    Convergent Phrase   0.253   0.064
21. Partial Repetition/Word and Spelling   0.004   0.000
22. Total Repetition and Elaboration   0.405   0.164
23. Elaboration and Syntactic Revision   0.400   0.160
24. Synonym and Word Congervence and
    Syntactic Revision   0.471   0.222
25. Partial Repetition/Phrase and
    Elaboration and Simplification   0.009   0.000
26. Partial Repetition/Phrase and
    Synonym and Word Convergence and
    Elaboration   0.484   0.234
27. Partial Repetition/Phrase and
    Convergence Phrase and Elaboration   0.302   0.091
28. Partial Repetition/Phrase and
    Elaboration and Syntactic Revision   0.090   0.008
29. Partial Repetition/Phrase and
    Elaboration and Spelling   ---   ---
30. Partial Repetition/Phrase and
    Synonym and Word Convergence and
    Syntactic Revision   0.253   0.064
31. Partial Repetition/Phrase and
    Synonym and Word Convergence and
    Simplification   0.267   0.071

SECTION II:

ASSESSMENT AND DIFFERENTIAL DIAGNOSIS

6

The Standardized Assessment of Dysarthria Is Possible

Pamela Enderby

INTRODUCTION

The term "dysarthria" is used in this chapter in a restricted sense, to describe faulty pronounciation or speech deviation due to neuromuscular disorders (Espir and Rose, 1976). Despite this restriction, dysarthria is the most commonly acquired speech disorder. Unfortunately, little progress in the clinical management of this disorder has been made in spite of active research in the field over the past decade. It is possible that this is due to sophisticated technological methods of assessment used in research establishments that are seldom replicated in the normal clinical situation. The needs of the test designer and the test user are often different, with the designer imposing an erudite method which generally leads to the user moving away from the standardized design in order to work within the physical constraint of a clinic.

Therefore, the conventional method of assessment is one of description. This method minimizes test reliability, or sensitivity, and leads to inconsistent findings by different authorities. The value of identifying speech symptoms in the diagnosis of neurological disease has been recognized (Darley, Aronson, and Brown, 1969; Berry, Darley, Aronson, and Goldstein, 1974). However, the difficulty in differentiating these patterns, especially when assessment involves less-experienced therapists, cannot be underestimated. A standardized, reliable, and valid assessment technique that can be used by all speech therapists in a normal clinical situation is essential to promote more initiative in the treatment of dysarthria. We feel that such evaluation designs are possible, and the objective of this chapter is to describe efforts toward this end.

DEVELOPMENT OF THE FRENCHAY DYSARTHRIA ASSESSMENT

Background

In 1980, a protocol for this study was described with essential considerations for the development of a practical assessment. This first effort detailed that the test results should be easily applicable to speech therapy, that the test should be sensitive to change, and that it should be short and easy to use. In addition, the assessment should require minimal training to achieve inter-scorer reliability, and the results should be easy to communicate to other professionals (Enderby, 1980).

The most commonly used method of assessing dysarthria by speech therapists in Britain (U.K.) is by describing the disorder with either a mental or physical check list. Based upon this description, a report is written which outlines the various features of the patient's speech. In studying a number of reports on patients written by speech therapists from all over the United Kingdom, we discovered common trends with regard to the areas being examined. However, speech therapists rarely commented on features that were normal or nearly normal, making comparisons with follow-up reports difficult. Furthermore, a descriptive report undertaken by two speech therapists on the same patient bore different weighting on different features, so that one therapist might stress a particular area of speech difficulty or concentrate accurately on describing one behavior, whereas the other might dwell more on some other characteristic. Dysarthria reports from nine therapists showed that the main areas of their examination included oral reflexes, respiration, lips, jaw, palate, vocal cords, tongue, and intelligibility. In addition to this, some therapists included comments on posture and rate of speech. Some of these main headings were separated into finer groups so that the appearance, activity, and function might be described. However, there was less similarity between the sub-headings. In the examination of a dysarthric patient, the therapist apparently required the patient to perform certain tasks so that (s)he might observe and comment on behavior. Although there was a certain similarity about the tasks and the length of time during which they had to be undertaken, we observed that the degree of skill to be achieved varied quite radically.

DEVELOPMENT OF THE FRENCHAY DYSARTHRIA ASSESSMENT

Description

In considering the type and degree of dysarthria associated with certain neurological disorders, it is necessary to include a study of the relevant anatomical, physiological, and perceptual features to achieve an eclectic view of this complicated disorder. It is of interest to note that speech therapists and neurologists over several decades have described dysarthria in this multi-factorial fashion, indicating the value of a comprehensive approach.

In 1976, a procedure for the examination of dysarthria was established by seven speech therapists representing two English hospitals. This protocol was basic and simple, involving twenty-two tasks. For example, a patient was asked to say "oo-ee" ten times, measuring the time of the second attempt. Meetings were held between the therapists on several occasions, which led to amendments and an expansion of the procedure. Tasks were altered, expended, or abandoned according to practical and/or theoretical constraints.

FIGURE 6-1
Alternating Movements (Example of scale: lips)

Ask patient to repeat "oo ee" ten times. Demonstrate by producing ten segments in ten seconds. Ask patient to exaggerate movement and to try to copy the speed demonstrated. Note his second attempt. Do not say in unison. It is not necessary for the patient to use voice.

a. Able to articulate both movements in 10 seconds rythmically. Shows good rounding and spread of lips.

b. Able to articulate both movements in 15 seconds. May have faltering rhythm, or variability in rounding and spreading of lips.

c. Attempts both movements, but labored. One movement may be within normal limits, but other movement severely distorted.

d. Shapes recognizable as being different. Or one shape managed three times.

e. Unable to make any movement reccgnizable as representing either shape.

In 1977, the descriptions used by our committee of therapists to describe speech behaviors involved in the tasks were collected. Each therapist appeared to favor certain methods of description to differentiate behaviors observed in individual patients. Although there were similarities in grouping of characteristics, it was necessary for accuracy of recording that our therapists agreed upon what constitutes a "slow movement" or what "normal" responses are for certain tasks. For each task a rating scale was produced which defined what score a patient should achieve for the behavior observed. Thus, a rating score was given to each possible result of a demanded activity. These descriptions were continually amended until a consensus of the seven therapists was achieved. Figure 6-1 is an example of one such task.

Result Form

The result form is similar to a bar graph; the vertical axis is divided into a 9-point rating scale, and the horizontal axis represents the main features which are then subdivided into the various tasks.

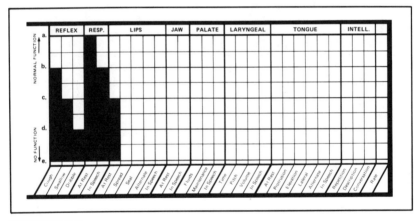

FIGURE 6-2
Result Form

A vertical bar is drawn to the appropriate point on the function scale to reflect the severity rating achieved by a patient on a certain task, so that upon completion of the assessment the pattern of the patient's disorder is clearly visible by a bar graph.

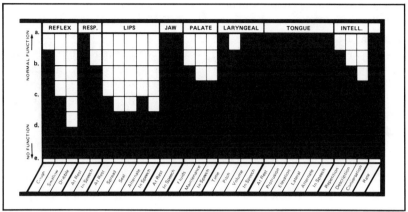

FIGURE 6-3
Result form in patient with lower motor neurone dysarthria

In Figure 6-3, the reader can readily determine that the patient in question has a drooling and swallowing problem complicated by lip and palatal involvement, which was measured on all tasks. Intelligibility, however, was only mildly affected, probably because there was normal tongue and laryngeal function. In addition, there is a place on the form to comment on extraneous factors that may influence the speech disorder or its recovery; for example, when there is a problem with dentures, or a hearing difficulty. Therefore, this method of recording results does not require transferral to a separate summary on a final report. This is further facilitated by no-carbon-required paper which enables the therapist to add comments and recommendations and then to detach the copy for immediate inclusion in the medical notes.

Normal Data

The first edition of the Frenchay Dysarthria Assessment was carried out on 46 normal, healthy adults ranging between 23 and 64 years of age (Enderby, 1980). The second edition, which contained revisions according to extensive clinical usage, was carried out on two age groups of normal subjects. In the first, 111 subjects comprised a young group between 15 and 59 years of age.

It was found that 94.6% of the younger subjects achieved a top grade (9), a total of 4.6% of subjects achieved a grade 8, and 0.5% were allocated to grade 7. Less than 0.1% scored lower than a grade of 6. If a subject scored the top grade on each of the 20 items, he could achieve a maximum score of 180. The lowest total score achieved by the younger group was 172, showing a range of 8.

A second group was made up of 37 subjects between the ages of 60 and 97 years. Analysis of the scale tasks performed by this older group showed 90.8% of the subjects obtaining the highest grade, and 8.9% obtaining grade 8. Less than 0.1% scored a lower grade on any of the subtests, results quite similar to those of the younger group.

Based upon these data, changes in the assessment protocol were made, but the majority of the items and subtests were retained. The main changes were made in ascribing scaled scores to certain duration limits in which performance on the assessment tasks had to be achieved. Previously, most of the experience of test use had been on pathological subjects; therefore, the top rating scale had been lower than it should have been to reflect normal ability. Thus, the test ceiling for a normal rating was raised for these items.

Interscorer Reliability

One of the most important dimensions for any behavioral assessment is that different judges will be able to describe the same type and degree of disorder in the same way. One of the main problems in standardizing a test is that the number of options of measurement available is inversely, but linearly, related to the degree of interobserver reliability. To achieve sensitivity and range of description, however, it is necessary to use as broad a severity scale as is compatible with acceptable interscorer agreement.

Eight speech therapists, who were unfamiliar with the Frenchay Dysarthria Assessment, had three hours' training in the test procedure. Following this, 13 video tapes of dysarthric subjects who represented a broad range of type and degree of speech disability were scored by these judges independently. In addition, three live subjects were examined by an independent clinician in front of the eight speech therapists who recorded their results.

The widest range of scores by judges on any individual patient was 15% of the overall score, and the majority of the patients' scores were clustered more closely. A product-moment correlation on each item between judges yielded high interjudge coefficients. See Figure 6-4.

JUDGE	1	2	3	4	5	6	7	8
1								
2	.79							
3	.8	.88						
4	.8	.88	.88					
5	.8	.89	.89	.91				
6	.79	.88	.88	.91	.91			
7	.8	.89	.88	.91	.92	.92		
8	.79	.86	.88	.89	.89	.88	.92	

FIGURE 6-4
Correlations between judges

Validity

Noted authors (Grewel, 1957; Darley et al., 1969; Thompson, 1978) suggest that certain features of speech are attributable to the dysarthria associated with specific neurologic disorders. The patterns of speech disability reflected on the Frenchay Assessment form were highly individual.

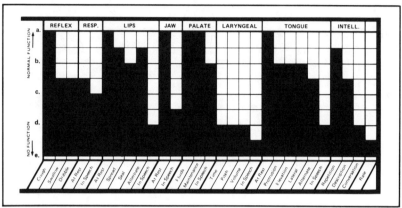

FIGURE 6-5
Result Form — Patient with extrapyramidal dysarthria

Compare Figures 6-3 and 6-5. The differences are obvious. However, the need to validate and confirm the differences was apparent. Therefore, to analyze which patterns were associated with underlying neurologic disorders, eighty-eight subjects with confirmed medical diagnoses were assessed with the Frenchay Dysarthria Assessment.
Their speech disorder was associated with:

Upper motor neuron lesions	30 subjects
Lower motor neuron lesions	10 subjects
Extrapyramidal disorders	18 subjects
Cerebellar dysfunction	14 subjects
Mixed upper and lower motor neuron lesions	13 subjects

In Figure 6-6, a discriminant analysis showed positive results for ability to differentiate the groups. The results of a prediction analysis were encouragingly high. Over 90% of the cases were correctly classified. Following this analysis, it was possible to establish the most powerful discriminating items within the test. It is interesting that four of the sub-tests, although reliable, were poor discriminators. These involved grading of performance on specific articulators within speech.

By removing these factors, the prediction results were improved to 94.6%. We decided, however, that these items should not be removed from the test in its final form, since the increase of prediction is minimal when compared with the loss of descriptive information in the four items, which are very useful in helping to plan treatment.

ACTUAL GROUP	PREDICTED GROUP				
	Spastic N= 30	*Mixed* N= 13	*Extra-pyramidal* N= 18	*Cerebellar* N= 14	*Flaccid* N= 10
Spastic	83.3%	3.3%	10%	3.3%	0%
Mixed	7.7%	92.3%	0%	0%	0%
Extra-pyramidal	11.1%	0%	88.9%	0%	0%
Cerebellar	0%	0%	0%	100%	0%
Flaccid	0%	0%	0%	0%	100%

90.6% of known cases correctly classified

FIGURE 6-6
Predictive Data I

ACTUAL GROUP	PREDICTED GROUP				
	Spastic	*Mixed*	*Extra-pyramidac*	*Cerebellar*	*Flaccid*
Spastic	86.7%	6.7%	6.7%	0%	0%
Mixed	0%	92.3%	0%	0%	7.7%
Extra-pyramidal	0%	0%	100%	0%	0%
Cerebellar	0%	0%	0%	100%	0%
Flaccid	0%	0%	0%	0%	100%

94.6% of known cases correctly classified

FIGURE 6-7
Predictive Data II

DISCUSSION

The Frenchay Dysarthria Assessment has taken six years to evolve, and it is still developing. One of its main strengths is that it was developed in a normal clinical situation. Therefore, all modifications were prompted by reality, so that our theoretical framework for test standardization led to the establishment of a useful tool.

We use this standardized evaluation procedure to promote a high degree of interjudge agreement within our clinic. As our data suggest, it also promotes accuracy of description and classification of the various types of dysarthria. Of course, there are constraints in using a standardized procedure. However, we feel that the issues of reliability and standardized description far outweigh the loss of test flexibility.

Beyond the obvious direct applications of the Frenchay Assessment in the clinical management of dysarthric speakers, it will also play a valuable role in training inexperienced therapists or students. Perceptual evaluation skills are at the very heart of the assessment of patients who suffer from motor speech disorders; however, learning to reliably listen, rate, and synthesize a list of speech characteristics into an accurate classification (i.e., differential diagnosis) is a formidable task. The Frenchay Dysarthria Assessment could certainly decrease the amount of trial and error time in this learning process.

Finally, since our test is reliable in rating the severity of dysarthric speech across a wide range of tasks, it holds promise as a clinical research tool. Unfortunately, most speech therapists do not involve themselves in single-subject research with dysarthric subjects because they do not have a standardized, reliable measurement instrument to determine the efficacy of their work. Our assessment technique could, therefore, provide a vehicle to improved clinical research in this area.

GLOSSARY

Cerebellar dysfunction — Confirmed lesions in cerebellar area causing ataxic symptoms.

Discriminant analysis — This is a statistical technique which produces a series of linear combinations (called factors) of original variables in a manner that members belonging to one (diagnostic) group have significantly different values of these factors than those belonging to other groups.

Extrapyramidal dysarthria — Motor speech disorder involving extrapyramidal motor system dysfunction, of which Parkinson's disease was the presenting disorder in this study.

Lower motor neurone lesions — Confirmed lesions of one or more lower motor neurones causing flaccidity of affected muscles.

Mixed upper/lower motor neurone lesions — Confirmed cases of amyotrophic lateral sclerosis with symptoms indicating upper and lower motor neurone dysfunction.

Upper motor neurone lesions — Confirmed lesions of upper motor neurones causing spasticity of affected muscles.

REFERENCES

Berry, W., Darley, F., Aronson, A., & Goldstein, A. Dysarthria in Wilson's Disease. *Journal of Speech and Hearing Research*, 1974, *17*, 169-183.

Darley, F., Aronson, A., & Brown, J. Differential diagnostic patterns of dysarthria. *Journal of Speech and Hearing Research*, 1969, *12*, 246-269.

Enderby, P. Frenchay dysarthria assessment. *British Journal of Disorders of Communication*, 1980, *15*, 165-173.

Espir, M., & Rose, C. *The basic neurology of speech.* London: Blackwell Scientific Publications, 1976.

Grewel, F. Classification of dysarthria. *Acta Psychiatrica Neurology Scandinavica*, 1957, *23*, 325-337.

Thompson, A. A clinical rating scale of speech dysfunction of Parkinson's disease. *South African Journal of Communicative Disorders*, 1978, *25*, 39-52.

ACKNOWLEDGEMENTS

This research was made possible by the generous support of the Chest, Heart and Stroke Association, U.K.

The author would like to thank Dr. M. Campbell, Professor A. Read, and Mr. A. Hughes, Bristol University, for their guidance and encouragement.

7

The Results of Acoustic and Perceptual Assessment of Two Types of Dysarthria

Christy L. Ludlow
Celia J. Bassich

INTRODUCTION

When faced with dysarthric patients, speech pathologists have the awesome task of assessing complex patterns of neuromotor disturbance embedded in speech expression. The movement disorder is usually complex, rather than due to a specific muscle paralysis. Many dysarthrias are associated with basal ganglia and/or cerebellar pathologies which disturb the initiation, temporal organization, rate, and accuracy of movement patterns rather than the muscle strength (Yahr, 1976).

Speech production in a normal adult has become an automatized skill, after undergoing many years of gradual refinement during speech articulation development. As an automatized skill in the normal adult, speech is fast, automatic, and contains consistent sequences of action. The dysarthric adult exhibits disturbance of these automatized skills due to a complex movement control disorder. Since the adult is no longer acquiring speech articulation skills, the role of feedback may be negligible in speech production and, thus, the patient may be unable to effectively alter his speech pattern. Assessment, therefore, must identify and quantify the alterations in speech movement patterns that are due to motor control disturbances. Because the patterns of movement control are disturbed, the integrity of the oral mechanism, its structure, and muscular components are not predictive of the patient's speech production impairment. Walking is no more the direct result of the strength of the biceps femoris than speech impairment can be directly reflected by the strength of contraction of the obicularis oris.

For these reasons, many have used perceptual judgments of the degree and type of impairment exhibited by patients during connected speech for assessing dysarthria (Darley, Aronson, and Brown, 1969a and b; Logemann, Fisher, Boshes, and Blonsky, 1978). Some perceptual systems, however, have limited analytic power for determining which aspects of speech motor patterning are affected. For example, the term "imprecise consonants" does not identify whether a patient's speech articulation is difficult to understand because of inaccurate tongue placement, or because of inaccurate voice onset times for producing unvoiced consonants. Further, perceptual judgments are difficult to standardize over time and across different settings, preventing the maintenance of adequate inter-rater and intra-rater reliability. Perceptual rating systems are also difficult to replicate, limiting the comparability of different investigators' results.

Some of these problems can be avoided by acoustic analysis and measurement of the speech signal (Canter, 1963; Lehiste, 1965). To standardize speech assessment, tasks assessing patients' speech production capabilities, as well as their imitation of more natural speech, can be recorded and then analyzed from sound spectrographs and graphic level recordings.

However, although the acoustic analysis of speech can be objective and reliable, it may not have the same degree of content validity for assessing a patient's communicative impairment that listeners' perceptual ratings do. That is, the acoustic measures may not assess those aspects of speech production that are important for a patient to be able to communicate accurately with others. Therefore, our purpose was to determine whether acoustic measures of the speech of dysarthric patients differentiated their pattern of impairment from normal in the same way as perceptual ratings of the same speakers.

Two groups of patients with neuropathology at different levels in the nervous system were selected for comparison with normal speakers, using two different methods of assessment; (a) perceptual analyses of speech characteristics by trained listeners (after Darley, Aronson, and Brown, 1969a, b) and (b) measures of speech production from spectrographic and graphic level recordings. The objective was, first, to evaluate the sensitivity of each assessment system to speech impairment by comparing one type of neuropathology with normal and, second, to determine the pattern of speech deficits identified by each system in two groups with different neuropathologies. By examining the speech symptoms identified as impaired by each assessment system, conclusions could be made about the usefulness of each system for examining various aspects of speech production when affected by neurological disease.

METHODS

Subjects

Two groups of patients were selected to compare the patterns of dysarthria with neuropathology at different levels of the central nervous system. Shy-Drager syndrome (Shy and Drager, 1960) involves atrophy of several central nervous systems, including the automatic nervous system, and to varying degrees, the corticospinal, cerebellar, and the nigrostriatal system. Early in the disease, there is pathology of the pigmented nuclei, including the dorsal motor nucleus of the vagus (Vanderhagen, Perier, and Sternon, 1971). In contrast, Parkinson's disease involves the substantia nigra, the locus ceruleus, and the dorsal nucleus of the vagus (Barbeau, 1976).

Seven consecutive patients who met the criteria for diagnosis of Shy-Drager syndrome with CNS defects were included in this investigation. All had signs of flaccidity in their oral and facial musculature, paresis of laryngeal abduction on fiberoptic nasopharyngolaryngoscopy, and upper motor symptoms. None of the subjects was receiving medication at the time of testing. Four of the patients were male, three female, with a group mean age of 60.0, ranging from 53 to 67 years.

Seven patients with idiopathic Parkinson's disease, currently receiving relatively low dosages of levodopa and carbidopa (sinemet), were selected to match the Shy-Drager patients in sex and within one year of age. None had signs of dyskinesia and all were clearly hypokinetic with tremor and rigidity when their speech was recorded. All were ambulatory, had bilateral movement problems, and complained of speech difficulties.

Normal controls with no history of neurologic, otolaryngologic, or speech and language disorders were selected to match the patients in both groups in sex and within one year of age.

Speech Recordings

Subjects were recorded in a sound-treated environment with a head-held Electret condensor microphone at a constant mouth-to-microphone distance of 7 inches. A 1000 Hz calibration tone was read at the face of the subject's microphone with a General Radio Sound Level Meter. An instruction tape provided the following speech items for imitation:

Extended phonation of the vowels /a/ and /i/; imitation of the same sentence at regular and fast rates; rapid repetition for 10 seconds of the vowels /a/, /i/, /iu/ and /ua/ and the syllables /pa/, /ta/, /ka/, /pa ta/, and /pa ka/; producing a sound or syllable as rapidly as possible after a click; imitation of a low to high pitch on the vowel /a/; imitation of pitch contours in two sentences; imitation of the vowel /a/ and the word /no/ at four loudness levels — soft, normal, loud, and shout; and imitating the following sentences with word boundary contrasts:

"It was a blue bell."
"It was a bluebell."
"They will sail boats."
"They were sailboats."
"She said a cross word."
"She did a crossword."

Perceptual assessment — Nineteen different speech attributes reported by Darley, Aronson, and Brown (1975) to be impaired in hypokinetic dysarthria and other speech motor disorders associated with basal ganglia disease, were selected for this study. An additional parameter, frequently noted in neuropathologies of speech, "glottal fry," was added. Definitions for each attribute were developed (see Appendix A) as well as the rating scales for each. Seventeen of the attributes were rated between one and seven. One represented no abnormality, two represented mild and inconsistent (occurring less than 75% of the time), three was moderate and inconsistent, four was mild and consistent (occurring more than 75% of the time), five was moderate and consistent, six was severe and consistent, and seven represented complete dysfunction. Pitch level, loudness level, and overall rate were judged on a 13-point scale, seven being the normal expected level, with one being the extreme on the continuum of too low, too soft, or too slow, respectively, and 13 being too high, too loud, or too fast. To provide a common reference for judging pitch and loudness, synthesized /a/ vowels were recorded with fundamental frequencies of 100 Hz for males and 200 Hz for females, and were played to listeners at 80 dB spl re .0002 dynes/cm^2 prior to listening to a subject's tape.

Three speech pathology graduate students participated as listeners. Prior to the study, 20 one-hour sessions of listening to training tapes of dysarthric and normal speakers were required to reach an inter-rater intra-class correlation coefficient of .85 or greater on each of the attribute rating scales.

The experimental tapes of Shy-Drager, control, and Parkinson patients were played to the three judges following training, with no information regarding pathology or normalcy. Listeners were two feet from a tape recorder in a sound-controlled room, with the playback level of the calibration tone set at the same sound pressure level at the listeners' ears as was measured at the subject's microphone during speech recording. The mean rating for each subject for each attribute was computed for analysis.

Acoustic assessment — The following methods were used to make measures of subjects' speech without knowledge of the speakers' identities.

1. The lengths of the extended phonations on /a/ and on /i/ were measured with a stop watch in seconds from the tape recording five times, and the model value was determined.

2. The peak intensity level in decibels re .0002 dynes / cm² was measured from graphic level recordings of the vowel /a/ and the word /no/, each produced at four loudness levels: soft, normal, loud, and shout. The intensity level of the calibration tone read at the subject's microphone face at the beginning of the tape provided the reference in decibels for determining the intensity level of a subject's productions. The range in decibels between soft and loud and between soft and shout was also computed.

3. The peak intensity level in decibels of the final word of four sentence productions was measured from graphic level recordings, with reference to the calibration tone intensity level reading. The speech intensity level for each subject was derived by averaging the four intensity levels.

4. The latency of speech initiation following a click was measured with an x-y digitizer from sound spectrograms. The distance from initiation of the click to the initiation of phonation was measured in cm and converted to seconds.

5. The total time for production of a sentence was measured from spectrograms. The time from speech initiation to termination was measured in cm and converted to seconds with an x-y digitizer for the sentence produced at a regular rate and for the same sentence produced at a fast rate. The difference in total time for the two productions was also computed.

6. From sound spectrograms of vowel and syllable repetitions, the following measures were made: the number of productions of a vowel or syllable in 5 seconds; the number of gaps in phonation (on-off phonations) in 5 seconds; the number of productions of a vowel or syllable in the first 1.5 seconds of repetition: the number of vowels or syllables in the last 1.5 seconds of repetition (4 to 5.5 seconds after starting repetition); and the number of repetitions in the last 1.5 seconds minus the number in the first 1.5 seconds (as a measure of change in rate).

7. Duration changes made by subjects in segment lengths and interword pauses, to identify word barriers, were measured from sound spectrograms. Six sentences contrasted the production of the same words either as two separate words or a compound noun in the same phonetic content. The distance from initiation of the first word to initiation of the second was measured with an x-y digitizer in cm and converted to seconds for each of the six sentences. The difference in time between the two-word (equal stress) and compound noun (unequal stress) conditions was computed to determine the degree of time contrast made by the subject to mark word barriers.

8. Measures of fundamental frequency (F_0) were made from spectrograms using a scale magnifier to expand the region between 0 and 550 Hz. Fifty and 500 Hz tones were used to calibrate the x-y digitizer. The F_0 contour was traced with the x-y digitizer cursor and read in hertz.

9. To measure mean F_0 in sentences, the peak F_0 on nouns in three sentences was measured and averaged.

10. To measure the change in F_0 with stress contrasts, the peak F_0 of the two separate nouns in the three sentences each with equal stress on both words was measured and the difference in peak F_0 between the two words computed. Similarly, the difference in peak F_0 between the first syllable and the second syllable in the compound noun was measured when primary stress was on the first word F_0 changes was measured by computing the difference between the two differences and dividing by the subject's mean F_0 in sentences.

11. To measure the change in F_0 during intonation contours in sentences, the F_0 at the high (H) and low (L) points on the intonation curve was measured as indicated from imitations of the following sentences:

Say(L) (L)that's(H) (L)ex(H)cellent(L)
No(L) (H)he meant(L) (H)you(L)

Five differences between low and high points in the first sentence and four such differences in the second sentence were both averaged and divided by the subject's mean F_0 in sentences to determine the subjects mean F_0 change in sentences.

12. The total range of F_0 on /a/ imitation ascending in pitch was divided by the subject's mean F_0 in sentences to measure the total range in F_0 a subject was capable of.

13. Two measures were made of perturbation in fundamental frequency. Mean perturbation was measured using a hardware and software system incorporating peak detection and conventional zero crossing algorithms to generate a voltage proportional to frequency, yielding an accuracy of 2.51 μ sec at F_0 equal to 100 Hz (see Ludlow, Coulter, and Gentges, in 1983, press for further detail). Mean perturbation was the sum of absolute differences in consecutive periods minus one, as defined by Horii (1979). Diplophonia ratio was developed as a measure of the occurrence of alternating periods of different lengths. This was computed by dividing the mean perturbation for adjacent periods by the mean perturbation for alternating periods (see Ludlow, et al., in press, for further details).

14. The mean F_0 on extended phonation of the vowel /a/ was measured at the same time as F_0 perturbation.

From these 14 acoustic analyses, twenty-seven acoustic measures resulted. The names and definitions of these are presented in Appendix B. These measures are grouped into five categories: rate control, fundamental frequency control, intensity control, stress control, voice quality.

RESULTS

To evaluate the sensitivity of each assessment system to speech impairment, the means and standard deviations of the Parkinson patients on the acoustic and perceptual measures were examined along with those of the age- and sex-matched controls. The means of the Parkinson patients differed from those of the normal controls by one standard deviation or more on 21 of the 27 acoustic measures (see Table 7-1). To test for statistically significant differences at $p \leq .05$, Friedman Two-Way Analyses of Variance (ANOVAs) by ranks (Siegel, 1956) were used. This nonparametric measure was selected because of the large standard deviations in the Parkinson patients. Significant differences were found on eight measures.

TABLE 7-1

Means and standard deviations of Parkinson patients and age - and sex-matched normal controls on 21 acoustic measures of speech production

Acoustic Measure	*Parkinson Patients*		*Normal Controls*	
	Mean	*S.D.*	*Mean*	*S.D.*
	(N = 7)		*(N = 7)*	
Rate Control:				
Regular Rate (secs)	3.27	0.35	3.90	0.77
Difference in Rate	.54	0.28	1.42	0.45
Latency /a/ Initiation (secs.)	.54	0.37	.37	.08
Voice Quality				
Diplophonia Ratio	1.21	0.37	1.42	1.10
Stress Control:				
Pause control equal stress	.86	.13	1.20	.24
Pause control unequal stress	.54	.12	.49	.08
Pause control change with stress	.08	.06	.20	.13
Fundamental Frequency Control:				
F_0 in sentences	176.4**	38.1	145.7	43.1
F_0 on extended phonation	163.9*	34.5	137.3	35.9
F_0 range on /a/	.67**	.31	1.66	.61
F_0 change in sentences	.30**	.12	.66	.15
F_0 change with stress (a)	.28**	.13	.45	.10
F_0 change with stress (b)	.28	.14	.35	.10

Intensity Controls:

Mean SPL (dB)	71.1**	7.41	79.3	3.68
Soft-Shout range (dB)	17.7**	5.8	25.7	3.92
Soft-Loud range (dB)	10.4	6.13	17.0	4.79
Shout spl (dB)	92.3	6.46	103.5	13.01
Extended Phonation Length (sec.)	18.9**	7.90	30.9	12.10

Voicing Control:

Vowel voicing errors	32.46	23.63	2.46	9.72
Consonant voicing errors	-.58	5.02	-2.50	1.35
On-off rate /a/	10.00	7.64	20.29	4.89

---

* χ^2 = 5.1 p = .02, in Friedman two-way analysis of variance
** χ^2 = 7.0 p = .008 Freidman two-way analysis of variance

The Parkinson patients had significantly higher fundamental frequencies in comparison with the age- and sex-matched normal controls in sentence production and on extended phonation of vowels. The range on fundamental frequency (F_o) was severely restricted in the Parkinson patients on vowel production, during imitation of sentence Fo contours, and during stress contrasts conveying linguistic meaning in sentences. Mean intensity level in sentences was significantly reduced in the Parkinson patients, as was their maximum range of intensity on the loudness imitation task.

Examination of the mean perceptual ratings of the Parkinson patients and normal controls identified 14 of the 20 variables where the means of the two groups differed by one standard deviation or more (see Table 7-2). Friedman Two-Way ANOVAs were used to test for statistical differences between the two groups at p ≤.05.

TABLE 7-2

Means and standard deviations of Parkinson patients and age - and sex-matched normal controls on 14 perceptual rating categories

Perceptual Rating Categories	Parkinson Patients		Normal Controls	
	Mean (N = 7)	S.D.	Mean (N = 7)	S.D.
Rate Control:				
Overall Rate	8.0	2.0	7.2	1.1
Inappropriate Silences	3.3	2.0	1.8	1.2
Variable Rate	4.0*	1.2	2.6	1.3
Voice Quality:				
Harshness	3.2	1.3	4.1	0.8
Wet Hoarseness	1.8	1.4	2.2	0.4
Strain Strangle	2.3	0.7	1.6	0.5
Breathy	3.2**	1.7	1.5	0.5
Stress Control:				
Reduced Stress	3.0	1.0	1.7	1.2
Fundamental Frequency Control:				
Pitch level	7.5*	2.1	4.8	1.7
Monopitch	4.2**	1.1	1.8	0.6
Intensity Control:				
Loudness	5.9	2.7	8.1	1.6
Uncontrolled loudness variation	4.0**	1.5	2.3	0.3
Monoloudness	3.9**	1.5	1.1	3.0
Voicing Control:				
Imprecise Consonants	3.5	2.0	1.6	0.5

* χ^2 = 4.2 = .04 on Friedman two-way analysis of variance
** χ^2 = 6.0 = .01 on Friedman two-way analysis of variance

On the perceptual ratings, the Parkinson patients had significantly higher pitch levels than the normal controls and reduced pitch variation in sentences. Further, the Parkinson patients were reduced in loudness, had less loudness variation in sentences, and excessive uncontrolled loudness variation. Differences in rate and voice quality were also found on the perceptual ratings. The Parkinson patients had a more variable rate and were excessively breathy in comparison with normal.

A second evaluation of the two assessment systems entailed the sensitivity of each to different types of dysarthria exhibited by patients with multiple systems atrophy (Shy-Drager syndrome) and patients with basal ganglia involvement (Parkinson's disease). Examination of the acoustic measures indicated that the two patient groups had mean values which differed by one standard deviation or more on ten variables (see Table 7-3).

TABLE 7-3

Means and standard deviations of patients with Shy-Drager syndrome and Parkinson's disease on 10 acoustic measures of speech production

Acoustic Measure	*Shy-Drager Patients*		*Parkinson Patients*	
	Mean	*S.D.*	*Mean*	*S.D.*
Rate Control:				
Regular Rate	5.08	3.36	3.27	0.36
Fast Rate	3.50	2.21	2.73	0.35
Difference in Rate	1.59	1.53	0.54	0.28
Voice Quality:				
Jitter Ratio	12.84	12.29	7.21	2.97
Stress Control:				
Pause control equal stress	.99	.26	.86	.13
Pause control unequal stress	.65	.22	.54	.12
Fundamental Frequency Control:				
F_o range on /a/	1.01	.42	.67	.31
F_o change with stress (a)	.11**	.26	.28	.13
Voicing Control:				
Vowel voicing errors	10.71	8.94	32.46	23.63
On-off rate /pa/	16.57	6.05	21.14	6.15

**χ^2 = 7.0, p = .008 on Friedman two-way analysis of variance

Only one of these variables differed significantly between the two groups on Friedman Two-Way ANOVAs. The Shy-Drager patients had reduced change in fundamental frequency on stress contrasts in comparison with the Parkinson patients.

Similarly, to evaluate the ability of the perceptual system to identify speech production differences between the two patient groups, the means and standard deviations in the perceptual ratings were examined. The means of the two groups differed by one standard deviation or more on seven of the perceptual categories. These are presented in Table 7-4. Friedman Two-Way ANOVAs yielded a statistically significant result on only one measure. The Shy-Drager group had a slower speech rate than the Parkinson patients.

TABLE 7-4

Means and standard deviations of patients with Shy-Drager Syndrome and Parkinson's disease on 7 perceptual rating categories

Perceptual Rating Categories	Shy-Drager Patients Mean	S.D.	Parkinson Patients Mean	S.D.
Rate Control:				
Overall Rate	4.9**	1.6	8.0	2.0
Increasing Rate	1.8	0.9	2.2	0.5
Voice Quality:				
Wet Hoarseness	2.9	2.0	1.8	1.4
Glottal Fry	2.2	0.7	1.6	0.7
Strain Strangle	3.4	1.6	2.3	0.7
Stress Control:				
Excess Stress	1.7	0.7	1.0	0.0
Fundamental Frequency Control:				
Pitch Level	5.9	3.1	7.5	2.1

**$\chi^2 = 7.0$, p = .008, Friedman two-way ANOVA

Both the acoustic and perceptual systems yielded few statistically significant differences between the two patient groups on these univariate comparisons. This was due, in part, to the wide dispersions among subjects' values within each patient group.

Because of the large within-group variance, the Friedman Two-Way ANOVAs which employ ranks to compare age- and sex-matched pairs, was used. The large within-group variance probably reflects the different degrees of severity among patients with the same disease syndrome. In dysarthria, patients with the same neurological disease syndrome often have different degrees of severity and will differ greatly on single-speech measures. Neurological syndromes are usually defined on the basis of the combination of impairments found together rather than on the severity of the impairments, since the latter usually changes with disease progression. Therefore, to differentiate between two groups of patients with different neurological diseases, their comparison on single measures is not appropriate. Rather, it is the *pattern* of impairments found in each group that is most useful for characterizing the differences and similarities between two types of dysarthria.

Discriminant function analysis is a statistical technique that can be used for this purpose (Bennett and Bowers, 1976; Ghiselli, Campbell, and Zedeck, 1981). Its objective is to derive a mathematical function that is a linear combination of several variables, each with a particular weighting, so that the resulting function provides the maximum discrimination between two groups of subjects. After deriving a discriminant function, the measurements made on an individual on each of the variables can be used in computing the value of the function for that individual which will identify in which of the two groups the individual belongs. Discriminant function analyses can be used either to test whether the combination of a particular set of variables will accurately discriminate between two groups of patients (the direct method), or to select those variables most useful in discriminating between the two groups of patients (the stepwise method) (Nie, Hull, Jenkins, Steinbrenner, and Bent, 1975). For the purpose of this investigation, therefore, stepwise discriminant function analyses can be used to identify the combination of speech variables that would be most useful for characterizing the speech production disorder of a particular group of patients in comparison with normal, as well as for identifying those speech symptoms most useful for differentiating between two types of dysarthria.

First, to identify those acoustic measures most useful for differentiating between the speech of Parkinson's patients and normal controls, a stepwise discriminant function analysis, Mahal method (Nie et al., 1975), was conducted, using all 27 acoustic variables. The results are presented in

Table 7-5. Eight variables were includud in the final derivation of the discriminant function yielding a Wilks' Lambda of .0027 that, when converted to a Chi Square, had a probability of less than .0001. Further, when discriminant functions were computed for each of the Parkinson patients and the normal controls, all subjects were correcly classified by the resulting functions, which included eight of the acoustic measures and their differential weights.

TABLE 7-5
Results of discriminant function analysis with acoustic data between Parkinson patients and normal controls

Eigenvalue	Canonical Correlation	Wilks' Lambda	df	p of χ^2
364.51	.998	.0027	8	< .0001

Variables Included in Discriminant Function

Variable	Weighting Coefficient
F_0 change in sentences	6.95
F_0 change in stress	10.59
Diplophonia Ratio	4.25
Soft-Shout Range	3.87
Fast Rate	6.16
Segment and Pause Length Unequal Stress	-2.14
Consonant Voicing Errors	-3.56
Maximum Intensity Level	-2.43

The eight acoustic measures most useful for discriminating between dysarthria associated with Parkinson's disease and normal speech were: reduced change in F_0 in sentences, reduced change in F_0 on stress contrasts, excessive diplophonia, reduced segment duration and pause length, a slower rate of fast sentence production, reduced range in intensity on loudness imitation and consonant voicing errors, and reduced maximum intensity level.

To identify which perceptual rating categories were most useful for differentiating between hypokinetic dysarthria and normal speech, a stepwise discriminant function analysis (Mahal method) was conducted, using the mean judge ratings on each perceptual rating category for subjects in the Parkinson and normal control groups. The results are presented in Table 7-6.

TABLE 7-6

Results of discriminant function analysis with perceptual data between Parkinson patients and normal controls

Eigenvalue	Canonical Correlation	Wilks' Lambda	df	p of χ^2
1066.13	.999	.00094	10	< .0001

Variables Included in Discriminant Function

Variable	Weighting Coefficient
Monopitch	16.36
Nasality	-31.08
Uncontrolled Pitch Variation	28.84
Imprecise Consonants	26.24
Wet Hoarseness	-6.16
Inappropriate Silences	-7.29
Excess Stress	-5.10
Uncontrolled Loudness Variation	-14.91
Variable Rate	1.82
Overall Loudness	-1.16

Ten perceptual variables were most useful for differentiating between normal and hypokinetic dysarthria. The resulting discriminant function yielded a Wilks Lambda of .00094 which, when converted to a Chi Square, had a probability of less than .0001. All the Parkinson's disease patients and the normal controls were correctly classified on the basis of functions computed using their perceptual ratings. Thus, the perceptual categories most useful for differentiating between hypokinetic dysarthric speech and normal speech were: reduced variation in loudness, increased nasality, uncontrolled pitch variation, imprecise consonants, increased wet hoarseness, inappropriate silences, excess stress, uncontrolled loudness variation, variable rate, and reduced loudness.

To identify the acoustic measures important for differential diagnosis between the two types of dsyarthria, a stepwise discriminant function analysis (Mahal method) was computed, using all 27 acoustic measures in the Parkinson and Shy-Drager patients. The results are presented in Table 7-7. The resulting discriminant function yielded a significant separation between the two groups (p < .0001) with a 100% accurate classification of subjects as Parkinson's disease or Shy-Drager syndrome based on the function computed with the nine acoustic variables identified in Table 7-7.

TABLE 7-7
Results of discriminant function analysis with acoustic data between Parkinson patients and Shy-Drager patients

Eigenvalue	Canonical Correlation	Wilks' Lambda	df	p of χ^2
475.39	.998	.0020	9	< .0001

Variables Included in Discriminant Function

Variables	Weighting Coefficient
Vowel Voicing Errors	-8.89
Difference in Rate	28.81
Mean Fo in Sentences	-25.63
Segment and Pause Length Change with stress	20.38
Soft to Shout Range	15.53
Consonant Voicing Errors	3.26
Voicing of Tense Versus Lax Vowels	10.70
Soft to Loud Range	-8.62
Segment and Pause Length Equal Stress	2.44

Six of these variables were more impaired in the Parkinson patients. These were: vowel voicing errors, the reduced change between fast and regular rates of sentence production, elevation of F_G in sentences, reduced voicing on tense vowels, increased consonant voicing errors, reduced change in segment and pause length with stress, and reduced segment and pause length in equal stress. Two measures of the intensity range were more impaired in the Shy-Drager patients.

A similar discriminant function analysis for the two patient groups was conducted using the perceptual data. The results are presented in Table 7-8.

The resulting discriminant function was also significant (p < .0001), with 100% accuracy in classifying patients into the two different groups based on

TABLE 7-8
Results of discriminant function analysis with perceptual data between Parkinson patients and Shy-Drager patients

Eigenvalue	*Canonical Correlation*	*Wilks' Lambda*	*df*	*p of* χ^2
628.00	.999	.0015	10	< .0001

Variables Included in Discriminant Function

Variable	*Weighting Coefficient*
Overall Rate	29.73
Uncontrolled Pitch Variation	-11.78
Monoloudness	15.84
Monopitch	-29.68
Breathy	30.93
Strain-Strangle	25.77
Wet Hoarseness	-9.63
Increasing Rate	6.09
Uncontrolled Loudness Variation	3.70
Reduced Stress	-1.23

functions derived using the ten perceptual rating categories identified in the stepwise analysis as most useful for discriminating between the two groups. The Shy-Drager group was more impaired than the Parkinson patients on all of the perceptual rating categories, with the exception of monopitch and uncontrolled loudness where the two groups were similar.

To examine the pattern of speech impairments of the two patient groups on the two assessment systems, Figures 1 and 2 illustrate the mean values for the patients with Parkinson's disease and Shy-Drager syndrome on the acoustic variables and the perceptual rating categories, respectively. For each patient, Z scores were computed for each acoustic measure to determine the degree of impairment relative to normal performance by the formula:

$$Z = \frac{\text{Normal Mean - Patients' Value}}{\text{Normal Standard Deviation}}$$

A Z score indicates the number of standard deviations a patient's score on a measure differs from the normal mean, and in what direction. Mean Z scores for the two groups are plotted in Figure 7-1 for each acoustic variable either found to differ significantly between the two groups, between Parkinson's patients and normal controls, or identified in discriminant function analyses comparing the Parkinson patient with normal, or comparing the two patient groups. Of the twelve acoustic variables so identified, the Parkinson's patients are more impaired on eight variables, while the Shy-Drager group was more impaired on three variables. The two groups were equally impaired on the measure of F_0 changes in sentences.

FIGURE 7-1

Mean Z scores of Shy-Drager group (■) and Parkinson's disease group (o)

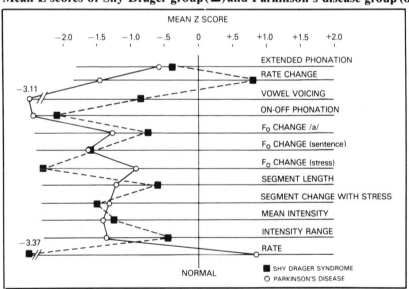

*On each of the variables in the acoustic assessment system found to be valid for differentiating between dysarthric speech and normal, and differentiating between two types of dysarthria.

The mean perceptual ratings for the three groups, the normal controls, the Parkinson patients, and the Shy-Drager patients, are presented in Figure 7-2. Ten of the perceptual rating categories were either found to differ significantly between Parkinson patients and normal controls, differ significantly between the two patient groups, or were identified in the discriminant function analysis between the Parkinson patients and the normal controls, or between the Parkinson and Shy-Drager patients. In all these rating categories, the Shy-Drager patients were more impaired than the Parkinson patients, except in two categories where the two groups were equally impaired: monopitch and uncontrolled loudness.

FIGURE 7-2

Mean ratings of the Shy-Drager group (■), Parkinson's group (o) and normal group (▲)

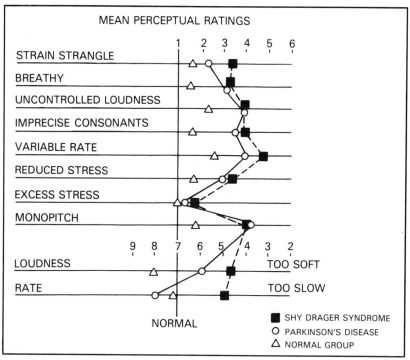

*On each of the variables in the perceptual assessment system found to be valid for differentiating between dysarthric speech and normal, and differentiating between two types of dysarthria

DISCUSSION AND CONCLUSIONS

On the univariate comparisons, both assessment systems contained several variables that differed significantly between the Parkinson patients and normal controls. Significant differences were found on measures of pitch level and fundamental frequency, the range in pitch and fundamental frequency, loudness and intensity level, and range in loudness and intensity. Thus, the differences found between normal and hypokinetic dysarthria in the two assessment systems were similar.

On the univariate comparisons between the Parkinson patients and the Shy-Drager patients, neither assessment system yielded more than one significant difference and the variables in the two systems were unrelated. Multivariate approaches were much more useful for differentiating between the two patient groups with both systems indicating that it is the *pattern* of speech disorder which is important for identifying the type of dysarthria, rather than the severity of impairment on any one particular measure. Therefore, for an assessment system to be useful for differentiating between types of dysarthria, it must be multidimensional, comparing patients on several different aspects of speech production. This was not necessary for differentiating between normal speech production and dysarthria. Therefore, single measures may be adequate for identifying when speech is impaired, but multidimensional measures are needed to determine the particular pattern of impairment.

Both the acoustic and perceptual assessment systems were capable of discriminating accurately between the two types of dysarthria. However, somewhat different variables were identified as most useful for discriminating between the two types of dysarthria in the two systems. Differences in rate control, variation in intensity level or loudness, variation in fundamental frequency or pitch, and reduced stress variation were identified in both systems. The acoustic system identified vowel-voicing errors as particularly important for distinguishing between the types of dysarthria, while the perceptual system identified differences in voice quality and overall rate as being particularly important. The additional variables identified by each of the systems may reflect those aspects of speech production that each system is better able to measure. The acoustic system identified vowel-voicing errors, a measure of the coordination between phonatory onset and offset, and oral articulation as particularly impaired in Parkinson's disease. The only measure of articulatory accuracy in the perceptual system was the imprecise consonants rating which was not found to be useful for discriminating between types of dysarthria. The measure of vowel and consonant-voicing errors in the acoustic system may be more specific to the speech articulation problems found in Parkinson's disease, while the imprecise consonants measure identifies any type of articulatory problem.

The perceptual rating system identified three aspects of vocal quality as useful for differentiating between types of dysarthria: breathiness, strain-strangle and wet hoarseness. Neither of the acoustic measures of vocal quality, jitter ratio, or diplophonia ratio were included in the discriminant function for differentiating between the two types of dysarthria. The perceptual system also identified overall rate as being particularly important for discriminating between the two groups. The acoustic system did not identify overall rate as being important although it did identify the amount of change in rate. It can be seen in Figure 1 that the acoustic measure of rate was impaired in the Shy-Drager patients in the same way that overall rate was judged to be excessively slow in the Shy-Drager patients on the perceptual system (see Figure 2). Thus, the results of the two systems were highly similar.

The patterns of results obtained with each assessment system are shown in Figures 7-1 and 2. In the acoustic system, eight variables were more impaired in the Parkinson patients, while three were more impaired in the Shy-Drager patients. As a result, the patterns of impairment for the two groups were quite different on the acoustic system. On the perceptual data, however, the patterns of impairments for the two groups are extremely similar with the main difference being that the Shy-Drager group is more impaired on all but two of the rating categories (see Figure 7-2). In performing perceptual ratings of impaired speech, the listeners may have gained an overall impression of greater severity of impairment in the Shy-Drager patients and given them more severe ratings on all categories. In contrast, the scores achieved on the different acoustic measures seem to be less related, both within each group of patients and across groups. Therefore, the acoustic measures may be more discrete for the analysis of different speech production factors in patients' speech. Further investigation is needed to determine if such is the case. If so, the acoustic system may be more suitable for assessing those aspects that are particularly impaired prior to treatment planning, while the perceptual system may better provide an overall indication of degree of impairment.

An additional advantage of the acoustic system is the separate measurement of a subject's capacity to alter a particular aspect of speech in contrast with his/her use of that aspect during speech production. For example, the range in F_0 in a nonspeech task such as the production of /a/ was measured separate from the range of F_0, during the imitation of F_0 contours in sentences, and during the linguistic contrasts between word boundaries. The latter two measures are indications of patients' use of their F_0 range, while the former is a measure of their capabilities to produce a normal F_0 range. In this study, the range of F_0 of the Parkinson patients was more limited than that of the Shy-Drager patients. However, the two groups were equal in their F_0 changes during sentence intonation and the Shy-Drager group was more impaired than the Parkinson patients during stress contrasts. These findings might indicate different treatment approaches for these two groups. The Parkinson patients had a high F_0 which, if lowered, could improve their capability of producing a greater F_0 range. The F_0 of the Shy-Drager patients, however, was within the normal range as was their capability for producing an F_0 range. It was their use of an F_0 range when making stress contrast that was reduced and should receive attention in treatment.

Similar results were found with the two acoustic measures of rate control. In one task, subjects produced a sentence at a regular rate and then produced the same sentence as rapidly as possible. The difference in time between the two productions was a measure of rate change. When making stress contrasts, the difference in segment and pause lengths used by the subjects when contrasting primary and nonprimary stress was measured. The Shy-Drager patients were able to change their rate of sentence production, while the Parkinson patients had severely reduced differences between the two productions. On the tasks assessing the use of segment duration and pause control for stress contrasts, the Parkinson patients produced shorter segments and pauses in the nonstress condition. Thus, both groups were impaired in their change in segment duration for stress contrasts, but possibly for different reasons. The Parkinson patients were producing shorter segments than normal during regular speech and could not markedly reduce their segment length on stress contrasts, while the Shy-Drager patients had normal segment lengths but, possibly, could not reduce their pause lengths due to their slow speech production. Thus, the Parkinson patients needed to lengthen their segments while the Shy-Drager patients needed to reduce their inter-segment pause durations. These types of analyses of speech errors — important for treatment planning — were only possible with the acoustic system of assessment.

TABLE 7-9

Summary of Acoustic and Perceptual Variables Found to be Valid* for the Assessment of Dysarthria

Acoustic Measures	Perceptual Categories

Fundamental Frequency Control

Mean F_o in sentences*	Pitch Level*
F_o in Extended Phonation*	Uncontrolled Pitch Variation
F_o change on /a/*	
F_o change in sentences*	Monopitch
F_o change in stress*	

Intensity Control

Mean spl*	Loudness
Soft-shout range*	Uncontrolled Loudness Variation*
Soft-loud range	
Shout spl	Monoloudness*
Extended Phonation*	

Rate Control

Regular Rate	Overall Rate*
Fast Rate*	Increasing Rate *
Difference in Rate*	Short rushes
Increase in Rate or Repetition	Inappropriate Silences*
Latency of /a/ initiation	Variable Rate

Stress Control

Segment and Pause Length Equal Stress *	Reduced Stress*
Segment and Pause Length Unequal Stress	Excess Stress
Segment and Pause Length Change with Stress*	

Voicing Control

Vowel Voicing Errors*	Imprecise Consonants*
Consonant Voicing Errors*	
Voicing on Complex Tongue Movements	
Voicing on Lax versus Tense Vowels*	

On-off rate /a/*

On-off rate /pa/

Voice Quality

Jitter Ratio	Harshness
Diplophonia Ratio*	Nasality
	Wet Hoarseness*
	Glottal Fry
	Strain-Strangle*
	Breathy

**Variables found to discriminate between normal and dysarthric speech and/or between two types of dysarthria.*

Table 7-9 is a summary of the acoustic and perceptual variables used in this research. An asterisk indicates those variables that were found to differ between the Parkinson patients and normal controls, or between the two patient groups on the univariate comparisons, or were useful in the discriminant function analyses, either between hypokinetic dysarthria and normal or between the two groups. Both systems had adequate measures of: F_0 or pitch level; change in F_0 or pitch level; intensity level or loudness; change in intensity level or loudness; rate control; and stress control.

The sets of measures where the two systems differed in their measurement capabilities were voicing control and voice quality. In the acoustic system vowel-voicing errors, consonant-voicing errors, and rate of phonation onset and offset were found impaired in both groups, and most notably in the Parkinson patients. The only perceptual rating category reflecting this aspect was imprecise consonants, which was not useful for differentiating between types of dysarthria. This may be because this attribute is not specific to the phonatory disturbances particular to Parkinson's disease (Logemann et al., 1978). For this and other types of dysarthria, more specific analyses are needed for determining which aspects of speech articulation are impaired. The distinctive feature approach used by Logemann and Fisher (1981) may be a perceptual approach useful in this regard. Additional measures of the coordination between articulators from speech spectrographs are also needed for the acoustic analysis system.

Finally, the measures of vocal quality contained in the perceptual system were useful for discriminating between the two patient groups. Only one acoustic measure of vocal quality was useful, the diplophonia ratio. Additional acoustic measures are needed for the objective assessment of vocal quality disorders found in dysarthria. Ludlow, Coulter, and Gentges (1983) demonstrated that measures of frequency perturbation are not reflective of vocal pathologies associated with dysarthria. Either additional measures of variations in the phonatory signal need to be developed, or acoustic spectral measures such as those developed by Emanuel and his coworkers might be used (Emanuel, Lively, and McCoy, 1973; Lively and Emanuel, 1970; Sansone and Emanuel, 1970).

To summarize, the results of this comparison of two types of dysarthria using acoustic measures of speech production and perceptual ratings of speech demonstrated that both assessment systems are valid for differentiating between dysarthria and normal speech. However, for both assessment systems, the differentiation between two types of dysarthria required a multivariate approach using a composite score of several measures, indicating that it is the pattern of impairment rather than the degree of impairment that is of importance in characterizing a patient's speech disorder. Finally, it was illustrated how acoustic analysis of patients' speech can be helpful in planning suitable treatment approaches.

REFERENCES

Barbeau, A. Parkinson's disease: Etiological considerations. In M. Yahr (Ed.), *The basal ganglia.* New York: Raven Press, 1976.

Bennett, S., & Bowers, D. *An introduction to multivariate techniques for social and behavioral sciences.* London, England: The MacMillan Press, 1976.

Canter, G. Speech characteristics of patients with Parkinson's disease. I. Intensity, pitch and duration. *Journal of Speech and Hearing Disorders,* 1963, *28,* 221-229.

Darley, F., Aronson, A., & Brown, J. Differential diagnosis patterns of dysarthria. *Journal of Speech and Hearing Research,* 1969, *12,* 246-269. (a)

Darley, F., Aronson, A., & Brown, J. Clusters of deviant speech dimensions in the dysarthrias. *Journal of Speech and Hearing Research,* 1969, *12,* 462-469. (b)

Darley, F., Aronson, A., & Brown, J. *Motor speech disorders.* Philadelphia: W.B. Saunders, Co., 1975.

Emanuel, F., Lively, M., & McCoy, J. Spectral noise levels and roughness ratings for vowels produced by males and females. *Folia Phoniatrica,* 1973, *25,* 110-120.

Ghiselli, E., Campbell, J., & Zedeck, S. *Measurement theory for the behavioral sciences.* San Francisco: W.H. Freeman and Co., 1981.

Horii, Y. Fundamental frequency perturbation observed in sustained phonation. *Journal of Speech and Hearing Research,* 1979, *22,* 5-19.

Lehiste, I. Some acoustic characteristics of dysarthric speech. *Bibl. Phonetica,* Fasc. 2. Basel: S. Karger, 1965.

Lively, M., & Emanuel, F. Spectral noise levels and roughness severity ratings for normal and simulated rough vowels produced by adult females. *Journal of Speech and Hearing Research,* 1970, *13,* 503-517.

Logemann, J., Fisher, H., Boshes, B., & Blonsky, E. Frequency and cooccurrence of vocal tract dysfunctions in speech of a large sample of Parkinson's patients. *Journal of Speech and Hearing Disorders,* 1978, *43,* 47-57.

Logemann J., & Fisher, H. Vocal tract control in Parkinson's disease: Phonetic feature analysis of misarticulations. *Journal of Speech and Hearing Disorders,* 1981, 46 348-352.

Ludlow, C., Coulter, D., & Gentges, F. The differential sensitivity of frequency perturbation to laryngeal neoplasms and neuropathologies. In D. Bless & J. Abbs (Eds.), *Vocal fold physiology.* San Diego: College-Hill Press, 1983.

Nie, N., Hull, C., Jenkins, J., Steinbrenner, K., & Bent, D. *Statistical package for the social sciences* (2nd ed.). New York: McGraw-Hill Book Co., 1975.

Sansone, F., & Emanuel, F. Spectral noise levels and roughness severity for normal and simulated rough vowels produced by adult males. *Journal of Speech and Hearing Research*, 1970, *13*, 489-502.

Shy, G., & Drager, G. A neurological syndrome associated with orthostatic hypotension: A clinical-pathologic study. *Archives of Neurology*, 1960, *2*, 511-527.

Siegel, S. *Nonparametric statistics for the behavioral sciences.* New York: McGraw-Hill Book Co., 1956.

Vanderhagen, J., Perier, O., & Sternon, J. Pathological findings in idiopathic orthostatic hypotension: Its relationship to Parkinson's disease. *Archives of Neurology,* 1971, *24*, 503-510.

Yahr, M. (Ed.). *The basal ganglia.* New York: Raven Press, 1976.

APPENDIX A

Definitions of Perceptual Rating Categories

Name of Attribute	Definition of Attribute

Rate Control:

Overall Rate	Rate of speech is abnormally slow or too rapid
Increasing Rate	Rate becomes increasingly fast within connected speech
Short Rushes	There are short rushes of speech separated by pauses
Inappropriate Silences	There are inappropriate silent intervals
Variable Rate	Rate alternates between slow and fast

Voice Quality:

Nasality	Voice excessively nasal. Excessive amount of air is resonated by nasal cavities
Wet Hoarseness	Wet, liquid-sounding hoarseness
Glottal Fry (Diplophonia)	Bubbly, crackling low-pitched phonation
Strain-Strangle	Voice sounds like an effortful squeezing of voice through the glottis
Breathy	Breathy, weak, thin
Harshness	Voice is harsh, rough, and raspy

Stress Control

Reduced Stress	Speech shows reduction of proper stress on emphasis patterns
Excess Stress	There is excess stress on usually unstressed parts of speech

Pitch Control:

Pitch Level	Pitch of voice sounds consistently too low or too high for individual's age and sex
Uncontrolled Pitch Variation	Pitch of the voice shows sudden, uncontrolled variation (falsetto breaks) or waver and modulation of pitch
Monopitch	Voice lacks normal pitch and inflectional changes

Intensity Control:

Overall Loudness	Loudness is either too low or too high in relation to a constant reference signal
Uncontrolled Loudness Variation	Voice shows sudden, uncontrolled alterations in loudness, sometimes becoming too loud or too weak
Monoloudness	Voice lacks normal variations in loudness

Voicing Control:

Imprecise Consonants	Consonant sounds are slurred, distorted, lack crispness and run into each other

APPENDIX B

Definition of Acoustic Measures

Name of Measures	Definition of Measure

Rate Control:

Regular Rate	Total time for sentence production at regular rate
Fast Rate	Total time for sentence production at fast rate
Difference in Rate	Time for sentence production at regular rate minus time at fast rate
Increase in Rate on Repetition	No. of syllables in last 1.5 seconds minus no. of syllable in first 1.5 seconds during syllable repetitions of 5.5 seconds
Latency of /a/ initiation	msec. between click initiation and onset of phonation

Voice Quality:

Jitter Ratio	Mean perturbation in fundamental frequency (F_0) divided by F_0 during extended phonation
Diplophonia Ratio	Mean perturbation for adjacent periods divided by mean perturbation for alternate periods

Stress Control:

Segment and pause length equal stress	Difference between initiation of two separate equally stressed nouns
Segment and pause length unequal stress	Difference between initiation of two syllables contained in compound nouns
Segment and pause length change	Difference between initiation times for equally stressed nouns minus difference between initiation times of syllables in compound nouns

Fundamental Frequency (F_O) Control:

Mean F_o in sentences	Average of peak F_o on six nouns in three sentences
F_o change on /a/	Difference in Hz between low and high points of an ascending vowel production divided by mean
F_O in sentences	
F_o change in sentences	Average of high and low F_O differences in sentence intonation contours divided by mean F_o in sentences

F_o change
in stress
(a) + (b)   Difference peak F_o between two words of stress
minus difference in peak F_o between words of
unequal stress, divided by mean F_o in sentences.
(a) is the F_o change for the words "blue bell" vs.
"bluebell," (b) is the F_o change for the word
"cross word" vs. "crossword"

F_o during
extended
phonation   The mean F_o during extended phonation of /a/

Intensity Control:

Mean spl   Average of peak sound pressure level on final
word of six sentences

Soft-shout range   Difference between peak sound pressure level on
"shout" production minus that on "soft" production

Soft-loud range   Difference between peak sound pressure level
on "loud" production minus that on "soft"
production

Shout spl   Peak sound pressure level in decibels on "shout"
production of the word /no/

Extended
Phonation   Length in seconds of extended vowel production
at comfortable intensity and F_o

Voicing Control:

Vowel voicing
errors   The number of vowel repetitions minus the number
of on-off phonations

Consonant
voicing errors   The number of syllable repetitions minus the
                     number of on-off phonations

Voicing on lax
vs. tense vowels   Number of voicing offsets with /a/ minus number
                     of voicing offsets with (i)

Voicing on
complex tongue
movements   Number of voicing offsets with /u-a/ repetition
                     minus numbers of voicing offsets with /i-u/
                     repetition

On-off rate /a/   Number of voicing offsets on /a/ repetition

On-off rate /pa/   Number of voicing offsets on /pa/ repetition

8

The Influence of Judge Familiarization with the Speaker on Dysarthric Speech Intelligibility

Kathryn M. Yorkston
David R. Beukelman

Speech intelligibility and related efficiency measures have been used as indices of dysarthria severity, as monitors of changing performance (Yorkston and Beukelman, 1980, 1981) and as aids in making clinical management decisions (Yorkston and Beukelman, 1981). Intelligibility scores are derived from a task in which the dysarthric speaker produces a message which is transmitted to a listener who in some way judges understanding of the message. A number of variables can potentially influence intelligibility scores and therefore need to be controlled when making clinical measurements. Some variables are related to the dysarthric speaker's task, such as stimulus length and complexity. Other variables are related to the transmission of the message, such as face-to-face, as compared to video- or audio-recorded samples. Still other variables are related to the listener or judge of the intelligibilty task.

A number of judge-related variables have been experimentally examined. In 1978, we reported the results of a study in which judges scored the intelligibility of dysarthric speech using a number of different formats, including transcription, multiple choice selection, and sentence completion. Results indicated that the rank ordering of dysarthric speakers was similar across formats, but that each format produced different intelligibility scores, with the highest scores associated with the sentence completion format, intermediate with multiple choice, and lowest with transcription. Another judge-related variable effecting intelligibility estimates is the judge's familiarity with the message spoken by the dysarthric individual. In a later study (Beukelman and Yorkston, 1980), initially naive listeners were progressively familiarized with the message being spoken. Results indicated that as judges became more familiar with the message, intelligibility estimates increased systematically for a sample produced by a moderately dysarthric speaker. In response to these findings, an attempt was made to control both judging task and level of judge familiarity with the message, using a procedure for randomly generating single word and sentence speech samples (Yorkston and Beukelman, 1980, 1981). The goal of this randomized selection process is to allow individuals to participate as judges repeatedly without becoming familiar with specific messages. Random selection of words and sentences from a large master pool is one means of standardizing the intelligibility judging task and controlling the level of judge familiarity with the message.

Still another judge-related intelligibility task variable is the listener's familiarity with the dysarthric speaker. In the clinical setting, listeners are often asked to judge the same speaker a number of times during the course of treatment. This repeated judging has the effect of making the listener more familiar with the speech pattern of that individual. The purpose of this study is to examine the effect of familiarization with the dysarthric speaker on intelligibility scores. Specifically, does increasing familiarization with the speaker, which occurs from serving as an intelligibility judge, increase intelligibility scores? If so, are the familiarity effects more pronounced for some levels of dysarthria severity than others?

METHOD

Speakers and Recording Task:

Nine dysarthric adults participated as subjects in this study. They were selected to represent a wide range of severity levels. Three were considered mildly dysarthric with sentence intelligibility scores over 75%; three were considered moderate with intelligibility scores between 40 and 50%; and three were considered severely dysarthric with intelligibility scores less than 20%. All subjects used speech as their primary means of communication and all had sufficient visual, language, and reading skills to read sentence material accurately.

Each speaker was audio-recorded as he or she produced two different speech samples. Both Sentence Set 1 and 2 contained 22 sentences (220 words). Samples were generated and recorded following procedures described in *Assessment of Intelligibility of Dysarthric Speech* (Yorkston and Beukelman, 1981).

Judges and Judging Tasks:

Nine normal adults served as judges and transcribed two speech samples from each dysarthric speaker. Judges were randomly assigned to one of three Familiarization Conditions.

No Familiarization (F_1) — After judging Sentence Set 1, at least two weeks elapsed before Sentence Set 2 was judged. No additional familiarization with the speaker was provided.

Familiarization with the speaker (F_2) — After judging Sentence Set 1, judges assigned to F_2 group relistened to the sentences in that sample *three times* so that they became familiar with the dysarthric speakers. Judges received no information about the message being spoken or the accuracy with which they had previously transcribed the sentences. Immediately after this familiarization phase, judges transcribed Sentence Set 2.

Familiarization with specific feedback (F_3) - After judging Sentence Set 1, judges assigned to the F_3 group relistened to this sample *three times*. These judges had an accurate transcript of the sentences before them as they relistened to the sentences. Judges were instructed to compare the accurate transcript with the transcript of Sentence Set 1 as they relistened to the sentences. Immediately after the familiarization phase, these judges were asked to transcribe Sentence Set 2.

RESULTS AND DISCUSSION

Judge transcriptions of the speech samples were scored for word-by-word accuracy. Measures of speech intelligibility (% correct) and rate of intelligible speech (intelligible words per minute, IWPM) were obtained. Mean intelligibility scores across subjects and judges for the pre- and postjudgings of each Familiarization Condition are shown in Figure 8-1.

FIGURE 8-1
Mean intelligibility scores across speakers and judges for three
conditions: No familiarization (F1), Familiarization with the speaker
(F2) and Familiarization with specific feedback (F3)

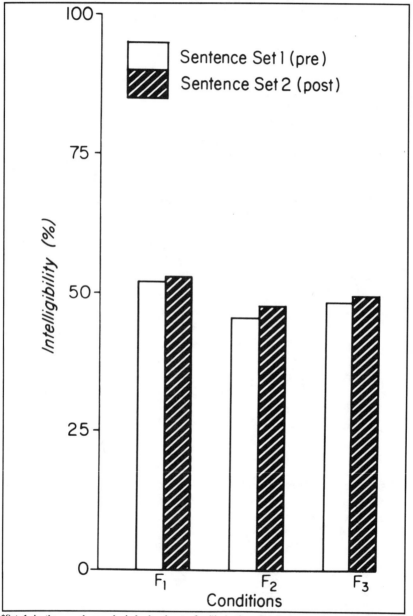

*Set 1 is the speech sample judged prior to familiarization, Set 2 the sample judged following
        familiarization.

These data were subjected to a two-factor repeated measure analysis of variance and post hoc analyses.

The first issue of concern was the equivalency of the prefamiliarization intelligibility scores across the three judging groups (F_1, F_2, and F_3). Examination of Figure 8-1 suggests that prefamiliarization intelligibility scores were greater for F_1 (52%) than for F_2 (47%) or F_3 (48%). Although the absolute differences among the mean prefamiliarization intelligibility scores were small, these differences were consistent enough to be statistically significant at the .025 level of confidence (See Table 8-1).

TABLE 8-1
Two factor repeated measures analysis of variance for intelligibility scores

Source	SS	df	ms	F	p
Total	47502.8	53			
Subjects	46320.3	8			
Familiarization	324.2	2	162.1	5.78	.025
Pre-Post	37.5	1	37.5	1.25	n.s
Fam. x Pre-Post	12.2	2	6.1	.81	n.s
Error Fam.	447.8	16	28.0		
Error PP	240.3	8	30.0		
Error Fam. x PP	120.5	16	7.5		

In an effort to explain these differences, the composition of each judging group (judges who participated in each of the Familiarization Conditions) was examined. Differences were found among the groups. F_1 was made up of three speech pathologists, while F_2 and F_3 each contained only one speech pathologist and two student clinicians. Evidently, the more experienced clinicians performed slightly, but consistently, better than the inexperienced judges.

The primary variable of concern in this study is the effect of familiarization on intelligibility scores. Comparison of differences between mean pre- and postintelligibility scores across the Familiarization Conditions revealed no significant differences with an F of 1.25 (Table 8-1). Thus, no familiarization effects were found for any of the judging conditions. These results support the repeated use of judges to transcribe intelligibility samples of the same speakers.

Figure 8-2 illustrates the mean rate of intelligible speech (IWPM) across subjects and judges for each of the Familiarization Conditions. Results of

FIGURE 8-2
Mean rates of intelligibile speech (IWPM) across speakers and judges for
three conditions: No Familiarization (F1), Familiarization with the
speaker (F2), and Familiarization with specific feedback (F3)

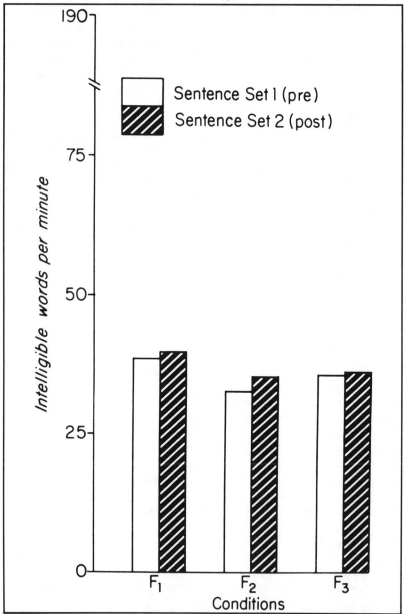

*Set 1 is the speech sample judged prior to familiarization, Set 2 is the sample judged following familiarization.

the analysis of variance and post hoc testing of the rate of intelligible speech are similar to those of the intelligibility data. No significant pre- or postfamiliarization differences were found (F = .6). However, mean pre-familiarization intelligibility scores were significantly higher for the experienced judges in the F_1 group as compared to the F_2 and F_3 groups. Because the two measures, intelligibility and rate of intelligible speech, produce similar patterns of results, the remainder of the discussion will focus on intelligibility scores only.

In the original analysis, the intelligibility scores were averaged across severity levels. No pre- or postfamiliarization effects were found for the total group; however, an interaction might occur between dysarthria severity and the impact of familiarization. For example, familiarization might have an effect on intelligibility scores of moderately dysarthric speakers, but not on the scores of severe or mild speakers. In order to see if this potential interaction existed, the dysarthric speakers' scores were grouped by severity, and the mean intelligibility scores were plotted for three speakers at each severity level — mild, moderate, and severe. The pre- and postfamiliarization intelligibility scores under the three Familiarization Conditions F_1, F_2, and F_3 are illustrated in Figure 8-3. Figure examination suggests no substantial pre- or postfamiliarization difference for any of the severity levels. Statistical analysis was not applied to these data because of the small number of subjects in each severity group. There appears to be no obvious interaction, however, between level of severity and effect of judge familiarization.

To summarize briefly, familiarization with the dysarthric speaker, even when that familiarization involved repeated listening and feedback about the accuracy of the listeners' response, does not appear to increase intelligibility scores. Further, some small but consistent differences among the judges were noted. Taken together, these two findings suggest that repeated administration and judging of sentence responses generated by a given speaker in order to assess the intelligibility of dysarthric speakers is a justifiable practice, if the same listener performs the judging task each time, and listener familiarity with the stimulus message is minimized.

At least one important issue has not been addressed in this study. We do not know if intelligibility scores are effected by the familiarity that comes with intense, daily face-to-face contact with the speaker, such as the contact a clinician may have with a client. It is reasonable to expect that such familiarity would elevate intelligibility scores. The extent of this increase awaits future experimental examination.

Thus far, we have focused on judge-related variables and their impact on the measurement of intelligibility. The implication of this and other research projects is that certain judge-related variables — for example, the

FIGURE 8-3
Mean intelligibility scores across judges for Familiarization.
Conditions when speakers are grouped by severity into Mild (N=3),
Moderate (N=3) and Severe (N=3) levels

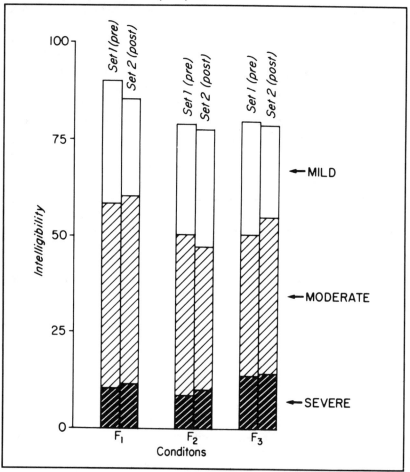

judging task as well as the judges' familiarity with the message—effect intelligibility scores and therefore need to be controlled as part of a standardized measurement process.

Traditionally, and quite logically, our treatment efforts have focused on the dysarthric speakers and attempts to improve the intelligibility of their speech. Intelligibility can also be modified, however, by changing the listeners' performance. In measurement, the goal is to stabilize listener performance. However, in treatment and in a natural communication setting, a more appropriate goal may be to maximize listener performance. It is interesting to speculate about whether or not listeners can be trained as an alternative, or a supplementary, means of increasing intelligibility, especially in the cases where completely intelligible speech is not a realistic treatment goal for the dysarthric speaker. Consideration of factors that maximize, rather than stabilize, listener performance would appear to be a clinically important avenue for future exploration.

REFERENCES

Beukelman, D., & Yorkston, K. The influence of passage familiarity of intelligibility estimates of dysarthric speech. *Journal of Communicative Disorders,* 1980, *13*, 33-41.

Yorkston, K., & Beukelman, D.A. comparison techniques for measuring intelligibility of dysarthric speech. *Journal of Communication Disorders,* 1978, *11*, 499-512.

Yorkston, K., & Beukelman, D.A. clinician-judged technique for quantifying dysarthric speech based on single-word intelligibility. *Journal of Communication Disorders,* 1980, *13, 15-31.*

Yorkston, K., & Beukelman, D. *Assessment of intelligibility of dysarthric speech.* Tigard, OR: C.C. Publications, 1981.

ACKNOWLEDGEMENT

This study was supported in part by Research Grant #G008003029 from the National Institute of Handicapped Research, Department of Education, Washington, D.C. 20202.

9

Bilateral Facial Paralysis in a Preschool Child: Oral-Facial and Articulatory Characteristics (A Case Study)

Anthony B. De Feo
Christine M. Schaefer

INTRODUCTION

Moebius syndrome is a rare disorder primarily characterized by congential bilateral facial paralysis and abducens palsy (Van Allen and Blodi, 1960). In many cases there is involvement of other cranial nerves (e.g., III, V, XII) along with such musculoskeletal deformities as clubfoot, syndactyly, or reduced muscle mass in the extremeties (Henderson, 1939; Merz and Wojtowicz, 1967; Rubin, 1976).

Until recently, the literature in speech pathology had not offered much analysis of the dysarthria resulting from Moebius syndrome. In 1971, Bloomer presented a discussion of two school-age children with this condition. A more detailed account of what they termed "congenital generalized bulbar palsy" can be found in Darley, Aronson, and Brown (1975). Two later publications (Meyerson and Foushee, 1978; Kahane, 1979) specifically addressed the speech, language, and hearing abilities of individuals evidencing Moebius syndrome. Meyerson and Foushee reviewed 22 cases and found that the extent of cranial nerve damage and corresponding degree of speech dysarthria varied widely among the children and adults they reviewed. Kahane's comprehensive case study of an eight-year-old male was carefully documented through an extensive battery of speech and language tests, electromyography of facial musculature, and acoustic analysis of speech productions.

The present case study offers in-depth observations of a youngster with bilateral facial paralysis. We will detail our observations and test results in profiling his oral-facial and speech characteristics at the time of our initial assessment (CA 3-6), and we will also present a longitudinal view (CA 3-6 to 6-0) of the articulatory adjustments he used in an attempt to compensate for labial paralysis. To our knowledge, this is the first account of speech and language behavior in a preschooler with this disorder, and the only case study that has examined change in speech behavior over time.

DESCRIPTION OF OUR CASE

At age three, our subject (John) was screened for communication and developmental skills in his local school district. Due to unintelligible speech and depressed scores on receptive language tasks, he was referred to the Idylwild Center for Communicative Disorders, San Jose, California — a self-contained classroom program for severly language-impaired children. Further testing was performed and he was subsequently admitted to the program. Curiously, none of the reports, including data from referral, initial assessment, or neurological evaluation, specifically questioned the possibility of facial paralysis.

John was then enrolled in a preschool language classroom where the clinician (C.S.) became increasingly concerned with his oral motor limitations. At that time, we (A.D. and C.S.) performed an oral-motor evaluation which led us to suspect bilateral facial paralysis. We completed further motor speech testing and reported our findings to John's neurologist who subsequently diagnosed Moebius syndrome.

History

John was born three weeks prematurely. He was described as unresponsive, jaundiced, and cyanotic at birth. There was a two-minute delay in respiration with cord loop noted. It was also reported that he displayed an abnormal Moro reflex and an inability to suck or swallow. At age three months, a tentative diagnosis of myotonic dystrophy was made.

According to the mother, John's early milestones were delayed until age 18 months, after which his motor skills improved rapidly and followed a normal sequence of development.

Characteristics at Initial Assessment (CA 3-6 to 3-8)

Oral-Facial Function: At rest, John's facial structure was marked by hypotonicity of the cheek and lip musculature, smoothening of the nasolabial folds, and an open mouth posture. Muscle balance was symmetrical and he showed no obvious sagging or atrophy. If anything, the cheeks had a puffy appearance. We noticed a slight downward angle of the corners of the lips. The description of 'mask-like' expression, often described in Moebius syndrome (Nisenson, Isaacson, and Grant, 1955), seemed to characterize him well.

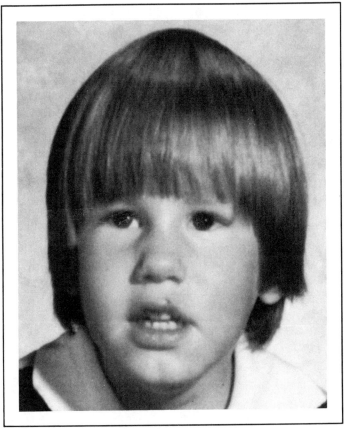

FIGURE 9-1
Reduction of labial retraction and elevation is illustrated during an attempt to smile

Figure 9-1 shows John attempting to smile. Observe the slight spreading—but no elevation—of the mouth corners, a characteristic referred to as "transverse smile" (Darley et al., 1975). His attempts to smile were accompanied by a forward thrusting of the mandible.

Equally striking was his performance on a variety of other facial function tasks. For example, he was not able to round, evert, or seal the lips and showed no resistance to labial manipulation. He could not imitate a frown or raise the eyebrows. During voluntary eye closure and eyeblinking. John's upper lids would depress halfway.

Over time, we did observe trace movements at the corners of the mouth, minimal elevation of the lower lip, and contraction of the neck muscles. In addition to these voluntary movements, we noticed involuntary, random twitches (fasiculations) in the lower face region.

In contrast to motor facial function, the symmetry and range of lingual and mandibular movements were much more intact. Also, sensation of the lip, face, and lingual regions was not impaired.

Examination of the oral cavity revealed an intact hard and soft palate, good dentition, and normal bite. At rest, the velum was judged to be slightly asymmetric (uvula tilted to the right), but range and direction of elevation appeared adequate during production of the vowel /a/. Active

TABLE 9-1

A summary of the allophonic substitutions and phonemic omissions noted at the time of initial assessment

TARGET PHONEMES	PERCEIVED RESULTS		TARGET PHONEMES	PERCEIVED RESULTS
Stops:			Glides:	
	p	ţ, k, ø, θ		w	wᴹ
	b	ḍ, g		r	ə
	t	t, ø, h, ?	Lateral:		
	d	ḍ, ?		l	o, j
Fricatives:			Nasals:		
	f	ħ, ө		m, n	ņ
	v	ḍ	Blends:		
	s	h ө		s + C	ħ + C
	z	h		C + r	C + ø
	ʃ, ʒ	ө	Vowels:	ɑ, æ	ə
Affricatives:				o, u	oᴹ, uᴹ
	tʃ	ө		I	Iʳ, ɛ
	dʒ	ḍ			

*Transcriptions were based on single word and connected speech responses.

movement of the lateral pharyngeal wall musculature was visible and the gag reflex could be elicited. Our inspection suggested a shortened length of the soft palate relative to the posterior pharyngeal wall, but we were cautious in ascribing significance to this observation.

We observed no swallowing or chewing difficulties. Interestingly, John created a seal with the tongue to drink liquids and to blow up a balloon. In simulating lip smacking, he produced suction by compressing the tongue blade against the hard palate.

Articulation — Table 9-1 lists the articulation errors we transcribed from his response to the Fisher-Logemann Test of Articulation Competence and an analysis of his connected speech. As expected, the place feature of labial phonemes was not attained. Errors among lingual consonants were also noted. Vowel productions were often perceived as lower or unrounded (probably related to lip and cheek flaccidity). Although from a developmental perspective we would not consider his productions of blends, affricates, or the /l/ and /r/ to be errors, the nature of these productions also reflected his physiological limitations. Intelligibility of connected speech was poor, with our estimates of initial samples yielding a rating of 25% intelligible with context known.

Voice Quality/Resonance — Clinically, evaluation of respiratory behavior revealed no unusual breathing patterns or discoordination of respiratory/laryngeal function. We perceived no abnormality of pitch, prosody, or rate. On the other hand, we and other clinicians did perceive moderate intermittent hypernasality, although he could achieve intraoral pressure necessary for apical stops, and with a model could sustain sibilants without nasal emission. John's nasal congestion contributed to occasional judgments of hyponasality and his frequent interdental tongue placements may have influenced our perception of a muffled vocal quality.

Other Assessment Findings — Despite the reported delays in language performance at time of referral, our observations and retesting showed normal language comprehension and expression. His reduced intelligibility made it difficult to quantitatively analyze a language sample, but within two months we established a Developmental Sentence Score of 7.52 (75th percentile for CA). Semantic relations and pragmatic functions were age-appropriate. The program psychologist determined his nonverbal reasoning abilities to be within normal limits, and a motor specialist assessed his gross and fine motor coordination to be at the four- and five-year levels of development. Hearing acuity was normal and the discovery of intact acoustic reflexes turned out to be a significant finding.

Discussion of His Neuropathology

Circumstances surrounding this case made difficult the use of a number of neurophysiological measures that may have validated our observations and helped better determine the nature and site of John's central nervous system involvement and resulting speech impairment. Two major limitations should be noted. First, instrumentation such as electromyography, biofeedback, or aeromechanical testing tools were not available. Second, John's neurologist decided not to seek additional neuro-diagnostic assessment since it was his opinion that such data would not have an impact on long-term management. Thus, we turn to the results of clinical tasks to summarize the extent of his pathophysiology and speculate as to the nature and site of the pathology.

Extent of Neuropathology — The primacy of John's facial paralysis was quite evident, yet we were initially cautious in ruling out possible paresis of other cranial nerves. The reported difficulty in sucking and swallowing during infancy suggested congenital, multiple cranial nerve involvement. Moreover, despite adequate lingual function on nonspeech, oral-motor tasks at the time of assessment, we considered the possibility that his imprecise placement among lingual phonemes, distortion of vowels and reduced ability to execute rapid lingual place/manner adjustments in connected speech indicated a mild hypoglossal paresis. This hypothesis was eventually dismissed when ratings and observations of his speech from age four through five consistently pointed to adequate lingual function.

Our perceptions of hypernasality led us to question the integrity of the velopharyngeal mechanism. Although visual inspection of palato-pharyngeal closure ruled out velar paralysis, we did not want to over-look the possibility that some degree of neural dysfunction was affecting the timing or range of velar movement in coordinated speech movements. Here, the use of cineradiographic or videoflouroscopic study would have been valuable. This was not pursued, in order to minimize John's exposure to radiation. Nevertheless, during the ensuing months of therapy we did not perceive the degree of hypernasality to be sufficient to seek further study, or alter our focus of treatment.

John's observed absence of eyelid ptosis and ability to abduct the eyes laterally pointed to normal function of cranial nerves III and VI, an observation confirmed by ophthomological examination. The integrity of trigeminal nerve V, which regulates mandibular movement and sensitivity of the face, was never in question. Finally, the positive results from examination of gross and fine motor skills ruled out other central nervous system involvement. Indeed, recent nerve conduction studies showed no evidence of a diffuse, subclinical polyneuropathy.

The uniqueness of John's condition can be appreciated when comparing him to other cases of Moebius syndrome. Table 9-2 lists various characteristics of some cases reported in previous publications.

As you read across this table, it becomes clear that the absence of additional cranial nerve involvement, especially C.N. VI, distinguishes John from the majority of other cases. Another notable difference is John's absence of musculoskeletal deformities, despite his early history of generalized dystrophy.

Regarding residual facial function, comparison among these cases reveals a tendency for the lower half of the face to be spared from total paralysis. For John, the degree of function in the lower face did not approximate that of Kahane's or Rubin's cases. Lacking electrical evidence we cannot be definitive, but our clinical judgments suggested some activity of risorius or zygomaticus, platysma, orbicularis oris inferioris and, unlike other cases, orbicularis occuli.

Site of Lesion: There exist two notions regarding the site of pathology in Moebius patients. One view is that nuclear or nerve agensis underlies the disorder (Van Allen and Blodi, 1960; Merz and Wojtowicz, 1967; Twofighi, Marks, Palmer, and Vannucci, 1979). Others (Evans, 1955; Nisenson et al., 1955; Hanson and Rowland, 1971) posit that Moebius syndrome is a muscular deficit, due to underdevelopment or aplasia of occular and facial musculature. Consistent with both these theories was Hanissian, Fuste, Hayes, and Duncan's (1970) intriguing autopsy of twins with Moebius syndrome. One infant exhibited hypoplasia of various cranial nerve nuclei while the sibling had underdeveloped muscle fiber. Such differences in findings, as well as their own autopsy studies, have led Pitner, Edwards, and McCormick (1965) to suggest two forms of the disorder, namely, myopathic and neuropathic.

In John's case, we knew from nerve conduction studies that at least the left facial nerve was capable of normal conduction. Could his facial diplegia be attributed to some type of residual muscular dystrophy? Perhaps his generalized dystrophy at three months of age had resolved in the extremities but not in the cranial facial musculature. Parker (1963) studied a family group of dystrophia myotonica and noted bilateral facial weakness as an early sign of the dystrophia. Unlike John, however, Parker's patients evidenced muscular and skeletal deficits throughout childhood.

The majority of clinical evidence pointed to brain stem pathology and John's unique response to a taste test further implicated a nuclear lesion. His taste discriminations were accomplished by placing the substances on the posterior portion of the tongue surface, bypassing the anterior two-thirds of the tongue from which taste sensation is carried by the facial nerve.

TABLE 9-2
A summary of selected characteristics of our subject compared to some other published cases evidencing Moebius syndrome.

	OUR SUBJECT	KAHANE (1979)	RUBIN (1976*)	MEYERSON AND FOUSHEE (1978**)
Number, Age & Sex of Cases	Male C.A.: 3-8 yrs.	1 Case - Male C.A.: 8 yrs.	8 Cases-Male & Female C.A.: 4 to 18 yrs.	7 Cases - 5 Males 2 Females C.A.: 2 to 19 yrs.
Extent of Involvement	VII (Possible XII & X ?)	VII V XII	VII (8) VI (7) X (4)	VII (7) VI(6) V (2) III (2) IV (1) XII (2) X(1)
Residual Function & Movement due to VIIth nerve innervation	Some Lower Lip Trace Mouth Corners Some Upper Eyelid Acoustic Reflex Neck Muscles (platysma)	Full Range-Lower Lip & Face Acoustic Reflexes	Some Lower Lip [7] Trace Mouth Corners [7]	NOT DISCUSSED Acoustic Reflex [6]

Associated Disabilities	NONE APPARENT	Malocclusion Submucous Cleft	Malocclusion (1) Mandibular Deformity (1) Extremity Deformity (2)	Malocclusion (1) Cleft Palate (2) Micrognathia (2) Extremity Deformity (6) Ear Malformation (1)
Other	Normal Intelligence	Normal Intelligence	Normal Intelligence (6) Mental Retardation (1)	Normal Intelligence (5) Mental Retardation (2)
Characteristics	Normal Language Skill Normal Hearing Normal Gross Motor	Normal Language Skill Conductive Hearing & Otitis Media	NOT DISCUSSED	Normal Language Skill (3) Delayed Language (4) Normal Hearing (7)

* Rubin discussed 150 cases but only presented the data on 8

**Authors reviewed 22 cases but only studied 7

Conversely, the discovery of normal acoustic reflexes seemed inconsistent with nuclear involvement since a branch of the facial nerve innervates the stapedius muscle. How could this be explained ? One lead is provided by Kahane (1979). In discussing a similar finding in his client, Kahane speculated that incomplete aplasia of the facial nucleus may have spared the cell group that innervates stapedius. He cited experimental data showing separate innervation of stapedius and platysma muscles within the ventrolateral portion of the facial nucleus. Might sparing of selective nuclear cell groups in the facial nucleus account for John's intact reflex as well as those reported by Meyerson and Foushee ? (See Table 2). At the very least, these findings call into question some of the typical inferences that are made (e.g., Jerger and Jerger, 1981) concerning the presence or absence of the acoustic reflex and the site of facial nerve lesions.

DESCRIPTION OF OUR THERAPY

John's enrollment in a self-contained preschool class for language-handicapped children afforded one of us (C.S.) the opportunity to provide articulation therapy three time per week. A description of the plan and rationale follows.

Since John's speech intelligibility was hampered by numerous phonetic substitutions and omissions unrelated to labial function, we designed a program of auditory-visual modeling to establish the place and manner features of /t/, /d/, /n/, /s/, and /z/. In addition, lingual patterning practice was carried out through production of phrases containing apical-velar contrasts, with John being rewarded for maintaining consonant accuracy while making rapid shifts across syllables.

Pretreatment analysis of labial phoneme attempts showed that he had not developed acoustically acceptable compensations. Therefore, it seemed appropriate to try to facilitate his use of articulatory compensations for /p/, /b/, /m/, and /f/. Our early efforts consisted of modeling labial productions and encouraging John to match their acoustic quality. Examples of verbal cues given are "use your tongue to make you sound just like mine" or "pop your tongue." Notice that we avoided detailed phonetic placement instructions so as not to confuse him or inhibit his spontaneous use of a variety of lingual adjustments, e.g., lingual-dental, lingual-buccal, tip-dental, etc. We believed it would be detrimental to his speech-sound learning if we imposed a predetermined, compensatory movement pattern.

As John began to acoustically approximate bilabial and labiodental consonants, we initiated a modeling program designed to emphasize his discriminative productions of labial vs. nonlabial cognates. A series of minimal word pairs differing only in place (e.g., me-knee, pin-tin) were modeled in a maximally different manner by varying intonation, volume, articulatory effort, and aspiration. Paradigms were established in which his spontaneous distinctive word productions had referential consequences, e.g., John produces "pie" and the clinician chooses between pictures of pie and tie.

Next, coarticulation of labials was drilled in polysyllabic words, phrases, and sentences. Practice in spontaneous speech was structured through story retelling, the content of which was phonemically loaded to include many labial targets.

Throughout treatment we attempted to increase John's awareness of his drooling and directed him to retrieve saliva with his tongue. We also encouraged him to maintain a closed mouth posture at repose. For this oral habit training, various monitoring and signaling strategies were employed.

OBSERVATIONS OF SPEECH CHANGE AND COMPENSATIONS

Intelligibility

Significant changes within the first few months of therapy included the elimination of /h/ as a substitution for tip alveolar stops and a reduction of consonantal omissions in connected speech. Vowel productions in nonlabial target words also improved and we perceived a decrease in hypernasality. Periodic articulation probes revealed that he was even producing affricates and some blends with accuracy. The sililants /s/ and /z/, while improved over earlier actualizations as /h/, were produced interdentally, and this pattern continued through dismissal from therapy.

In order to more reliably evaluate changes in John's speech intelligibility, we asked five listeners to rate samples of his spontaneous speech which were selected from our initial assessment, and at four month intervals thereafter. In editing these samples, we eliminated clinician comments that might have clued the listener to content or context. The audiotaped samples were presented in random sequence and the listeners (M.A. level speech pathologists) were instructed to rate intelligibility on a five point, equal interval scale with a rating of 1 denoting unintelligible and 5 intelligible speech.

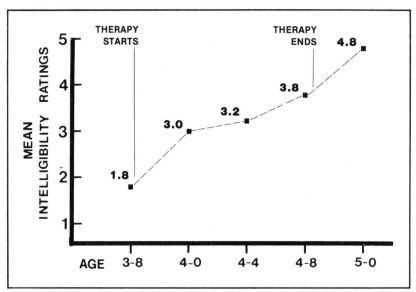

FIGURE 9-2
Mean intelligibility ratings of spontaneous connected speech samples by 5
listeners over the course of therapy and three months post-dismissal.
*John's age ranged from 3 years, 8 months to 5 years.

Figure 9-2 depicts the mean ratings of the listeners. Note the appreciable
increase in ratings over time. These data are consistent with our clinical
impressions and transcriptions of his responses.

Articulatory Compensations

Could a four-year-old child learn articulatory compensations for labial
sounds, and if so, what adjustments would he use ?

Between three and six months into therapy, John established a lingual-
interdental place of articulation for /p/, /b/, /f/, and /m/. Keep in mind
that we did not instruct him to use this place of articulation. Most revealing
is the fact that this placement was distinct from the lingual-dental
placement (tongue to upper incisors) he used for tip-alveolar targets /t/,
/d/, and /n/. Conceivably, this was reflecting his establishment of a
phonological place rule to distinguish labial vs. apical phonemes.

While compensatory placement emerged early in therapy,
approximation of the manner feature of labials was slower to develop. For

instance, three months into therapy nearly 50% of his /p/ and /b/ attempts were articulated with frication. It may be that in establishing compensatory place of labial productions he sacrificed manner.

At six months of therapy, the majority of his labial plosive attempts were produced as stops, although the acoustic result was often indistinguishable from apical stops. As we introduced contrastive production drills, John used two new behaviors to refine acoustic output. One adjustment was the insertion of a glottal stop between the target plosive and ensuing vowel. A second, more frequently used adjustment was an increase in articulatory force when producing /p/ and /b/ vs. /t/ and /d/. He appeared to anchor the tongue tip between his teeth and either delayed the release (for voiced /b/) or overaspirated upon release (for voiceless /p/). Possibly, this tendency to anchor the tongue tip between the teeth disrupted the anticipatory tongue posturing for various vowels, resulting in lowering of vowel targets. Also, recalling our earlier observation of hypernasality, we wondered if the lingual anchoring and increased force were influencing velar valving.

The final three months of therapy were marked by continual refinement of the acoustic quality of labial attempts. Additionally, we were encouraged by his response to oral habits training. John frequently retrieved saliva with his tongue and no longer displayed an open mouth posture at rest. One year after the initiation of therapy (CA 4-9), we dismissed him from our program and recommended continued therapy, as needed, in kindergarten.

PERCEPTUAL AND ACOUSTIC ANALYSES OF COMPENSATIONS

Listener Ratings (CA 4-3 and 4-9)

We first perceived acoustically acceptable labial productions at six months into therapy and at that time decided to sample other listeners' judgments. A videotape was made of spontaneous single words containing four productions of /p/, /b/, and /m/ and four productions of the place cognates /t/, /d/, and /n/. Two samples of /f/ and /θ/ contrasts were also included. His word productions were randomly sequenced and edited into a single tape. We asked 18 colleagues to view the tape and transcribe each word. For any phoneme, then, a maximum total of 72 correct (4 word samples x 18 listeners) perceptions could be attained. We repeated this task using responses he produced at 12 months into therapy.

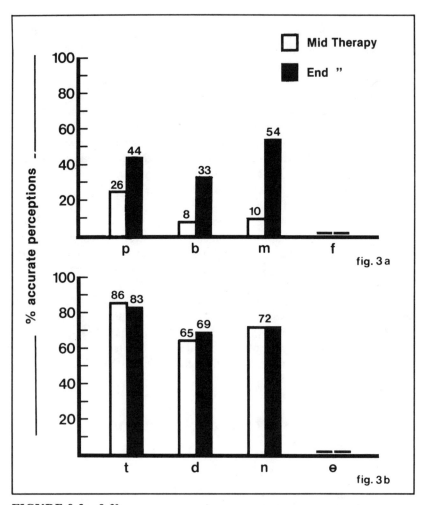

FIGURE 9-3a, 9-3b
Measures of phoneme accuracy at 6 and 12 months into therapy

*Figure 3a shows the mean percent of accurate perceptions of labial attempts and Figure 3b illustrates ratings of tip-alveolar consonants. Measures are based on 18 listeners' judgments of each phoneme produced in four separate words.

The percentage of accurate listener perceptions of John's responses at these points in time is shown in Figure 9-3a and 9-3b. As can be seen in Figure 9-3a, an increase in perceptions of labial targets occurred at 12 months, but even then the ratings approximated only 50%. In contrast, listeners perceived nonlabial consonants more accurately and with little difference at the midpoint and end of therapy. The listeners' virtual inability to discriminate John's /f/ and /θ/ word productions separate from context is not surprising when one considers the minimal cues normally carried by these phonemes.

In general, these ratings appear quite low but it should be pointed out that this was a stringent measure of phoneme intelligibility. Had these words been presented as contrasts or in meaningful context, we suspect the perceptions would have been more accurate.

Over time, we came to notice that if we inadvertently turned our backs to John or did not observe his face, we tended to more readily perceive acoustic distinctions between his labial and lingual phoneme attempts. To further assess this impression, his taped single-word productions from 12 months into therapy were presented to listeners under two conditions: 1) audiovideo presentation and 2) audio playback. The order of presentation of these two conditions varied among the 18 listeners. Their perceptions of consonants from audiovideo vs. audio samples were compared and the results are illustrated in Figure 9-4.

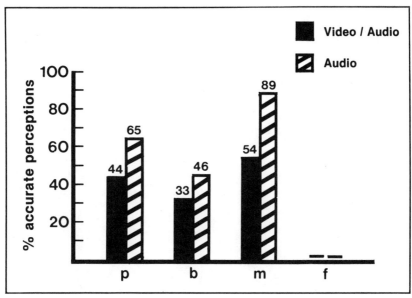

FIGURE 9-4

A comparison of 18 listeners' perceptions of phoneme accuracy, expressed as mean percent of accurate perceptions, under two conditions: audiovideo presentation and audio presentation of responses

*Responses were taken from samples produced at 12 months into therapy, prior to dismissal.

Note that the listeners perceived the labial targets more accurately when only listening to his productions, as opposed to listening and viewing. One interpretation of this result is that the listeners' observation of his visible lingual adjustments in producing /p/, /b/, and /m/ had a negative effect on their perceptions. Another explanation might be that absence of labial movement was the feature that altered their perceptions.

Listener Ratings (CA 6-2)

Very recently we had the opportunity to gather additional samples of John's speech. Audiorecordings were used to further assess listener perceptions of his labial targets and the results are extremely encouraging. First, we played a series of 20 minimal word pair productions to three clinical supervisors and asked them to phonetically transcribe each pair. Included in these word pairs were the place cognates p-t, b-d, and m-n. The mean number of pairs correctly perceived by these sophisticated listeners was 14.3 — approximately 75% of his labial-apical contrasts. Next, we obtained, through repetition, John's production of connected utterances containing multiple labial targets. Verbatim transcriptions of these utterances were given to 10 undergraduate speech and language pathology students and they were instructed to listen to each sentence twice and allophonically denote their perceptions of all consonants. Data from this task are displayed in Table 9-3.

TABLE 9-3
Listeners' ratings of labial phoneme attempts produced in sentence contexts

LABIAL TARGET	*# IN SAMPLE*	*MEAN # PERCEIVED BY 10 LISTENERS*
/b/	6	5.1
/p/	5	4.8
/m/	5	5.0
/f/	6	3.6
/w/, /wh/	2	1.9
TOTAL	*24*	*20.4*

æMeasures reflect the mean number of correct perceptions among the 10 listeners.

The intelligibility of his compensations can be appreciated be comparing the number of labial targets in the sample with the mean number perceived by the 10 listeners. In total, these listeners heard his lingual adjustments as labial productions 85% of the time. John had maintained, if not improved, his compensatory articulation ability during the school year.

Spectrographic Analyses
(CA 5-0 and 6-2)

Finally, we were curious if perceptions of successful labial vs. apical distinctions would correlate with expected differences in his production of acoustic cues. Audiotape recordings of contrastive words containing p-t, b-d, and m-n initial consonants were spectrographically analyzed from samples taken at ages five and six years. We examined these spectrograms for distinctions in two critical place cues: 1) the locus and direction of second formant transitions (F_2) and 2) the frequency of burst noise at the spike of the stop consonant. Figure 9-5abc displays three wide bank spectrograms that are representative of the trends we observed. Compare with the F_2 transition in each (designated by arrow 1). Observe that the F_2 transitions following labial consonants are characterized by a rising slope and originate at a lower frequency than the F_2 transitions following tip-

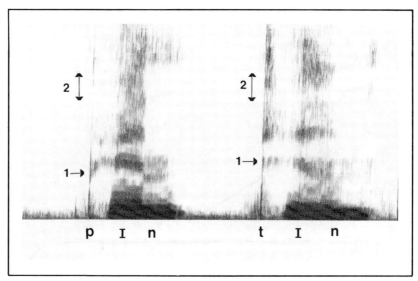

FIGURE 9-5a
Wide band spectograms of minimal word differing by place of articulation
*Figure 5a is pin-tin, spoken at age six

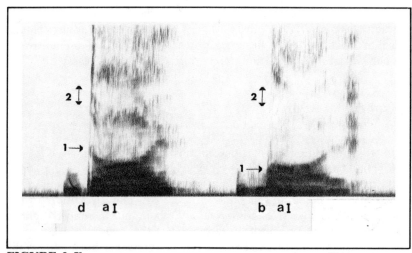

FIGURE 9-5b
Wide band spectogram of word differing by place of articulation
Figure 5b is die-buy, spoken at age five

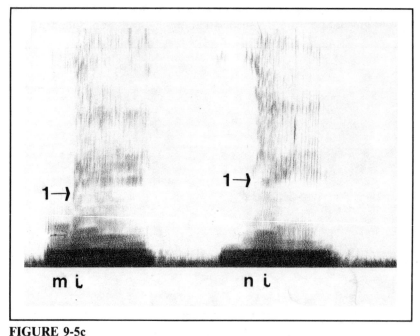

FIGURE 9-5c
Wide band spectograms of words differing by place of articulation
Figure 5c is me-knee, spoken at age six.

alveolar consonants. In Figure 9-5a and 9-5b, the greater distribution of burst noise in higher frequencies (arrow 2) for /t/ and /d/ vs. /p/ and /b/ can be seen. The trend observed in these and seven other spectrograms indicates that John's use of a lingual-interdental place of production (which, of course, lengthens the vocal tract compared to lingual-alveolar consonants) was an acoustically efficient compensation for the inability to achieve bilabial valving.

SUMMARY AND FUTURE CONSIDERATIONS

Circumstances leading to the eventual recognition of this remarkable child's oral-motor deficit re-emphasize the importance of the speech pathologist's role in carrying out a careful assessment of motor speech abilities prior to initiating treatment. Since we did not preplan a controlled single-subject design, no conclusions with respect to treatment effect can be made. Our clinical "hunch" is that intervention accelerated John's improved intelligibility; however, we acknowledge the role of maturation in this process. More importantly, considering the acoustic acceptability of John's labial phonemes at age five and six, we stand in awe of the compensatory capabilities of the speech motor system.

Would John have developed compensations for labial consonants without intervention? Many clinicians, including ourselves, have encountered clients who have spontaneously compensated for a host of oral-motor or structural deficiencies. Regarding Moebius syndrome, Meyerson and Foushee (1978) observed that some of their older subjects "used compensatory placement for difficult phonemes and achieved near normal acoustic output with these substitutions" (p. 361). Conversely, Kahane's (1979) and Shelton's[1] accounts of school-age cases indicated these children had not developed acceptable compensations for labial dysarthria. Because of John's age, we believed it appropriate to try to facilitate acquisition of consonant compensations. Keep in mind that our decision to provide therapy was also influenced by his use of aberrant articulatory patterns unrelated to facial paralysis.

In closing, there remain some future considerations which we will briefly addressed below.

Refinement of Articulatory Compensations

Since listeners' perceptions of phoneme accuracy were affected by John's visible articulatory adjustments, we wonder if in the future he should be encouraged to develop a pattern of lingual compensation within the oral cavity, much like ventriloquial speech. Some time ago, we had the opportunity to assist in the evaluation of a 14-year-old girl with Moebius syndrome who used just such an adjustment. Fisher (1981) is planning soon to publish a cineradiographic and acoustic analysis of this subject's speech pattern.

Social-Emotional Development

We suspect that John's facial paralysis might have an impact on his future social-emotional development. At age six, John told us he didn't like having his picture taken in school because of difficulty smiling. Recently, his first grade teacher indicated that he is experiencing behavior problems in school. Are these possibly the result of peers' and teachers' inability to read John's affect and mood? The inability to perform differential facial expression and function during primary and preadolescent ages could result in the development of a negative self-concept, and John may need guidance in learning how to express subtle pragmatic intentions through the use of vocal rather than nonverbal cues.

Medical Management

It is certainly beyond the scope of the speech and language pathologist to determine nature and extent of neuropathology. We took the liberty of such speculation in this report because it illustrated the problem-solving process we attempted to follow in making clinical decisions. We do think that further neurodiagnostic investigation should be pursued. For example, we look forward to medical opinions as to the feasibility of such corrective procedures as neural anastonomosis or muscle transfers (Puckett and Beg, 1978; Rubin, 1976). We remain hopeful.

NOTE

[1]After presenting this paper at the Clinical Dysarthria Conference, Shelton provided us a reprint of a case study he had done. Regrettably, we were not aware of this article (published in the *Kansas Journal of Speech and Hearing Disorders*) during our work with John, or in preparing earlier sections of this paper. His client was strikingly similar to John and the interested reader should consult Shelton (1963).

REFERENCES

Bloomer, H. Speech defect associated with dental malocclusion and related abnormalities. In L. Travis (Ed.), *Handbook of speech pathology and audiology.* New York: Appleton-Century Crofts, 1971.

Darley, F., Aronson, A., & Brown, J. *Motor speech disorders.* Philadelphia: W.B. Saunders, 1975.

Evans, P. Nuclear agenesis. *Archives of Disease in Childhood,* 1955, *30,* 305-311.

Fisher, H. Personal communication, 1981.

Hanissian, A., Fuste, F., Hayes, W., & Duncan, J. Möbius syndrome in twins. *American Journal of Diseases of Children,* 1970, *120,* 472-475.

Hanson, P., & Rowland, L. Möbius syndrome and facios ceapulohumeral muscular dystrophy. *Archives of Neurology,* 1971, *24,* 31-35.

Henderson, J. The cogenital facial diplegia syndrome: Clinical features, pathology and aetiology: A review of 60 cases. *Brain,* 1939, *62,* 381-403.

Jerger, J., & Jerger, S. *Auditory disorders: A manual for clinical evaluation.* Boston: Little, Brown and Co., 1981.

Kahane, J. Pathophysiological effects of Möbius syndrome on speech and hearing. *Archives of Otolaryngology,* 1979, *105,* 29-34.

Merz, M., & Wojtowicz, S. The Möbius Syndrome. *American Journal of Ophthalmology.* 1967, *63,* 837-840.

Meyerson, M., & Foushee, D. Speech, language and hearing in Moebius syndrome. *Developmental Medicine and Child Neurology,* 1978, *20,* 357-365.

Nisenson, A., Isaacson, A., & Grant, S. Masklike facies with associated congenital anomalies (Möbius syndrome). *Journal of Pediatrics,* 1955, *46,* 255-261.

Parker, N. Dystrophia myotonica presenting as congenital facial diplegia. *Med. J. Aust.,* 1963, *2* (23), 939-944.

Pitner, S., Edwards, J., & McCormick, W. Observations of the pathology of the Moebius syndrome. *Journal of Neurology, Neurosurgery and Psychiatry*, 1965, *28*, 362-373.

Puckett, C., & Beg, A. Facial reanimation in Möbius syndrome. *Southern Medical Journal*, 1978, *71*, (12), 1498-1500.

Rubin, L. The Moebius syndrome: Bilateral facial diplegia. *Clinics in Plastic Surgery*, 1976, *3*, (4), 625-636.

Shelton, R. Facial paresis and articulation impairment—A case study. *J. Kansas Speech Hearing Dis.*, 1963, *4*, (63), 2-9.

Twofighi, J., Marks, K., Palmer, E., & Vannucci, R. Möbius syndrome: Neuropathologic observations. *Acta Neuropathol. (Berl)*, 1979, *48*, 11-17.

Van Allen, M., & Blodi, F. Neurologic aspects of the Möbius syndrome. *Neurology*, 1960, *10*, (3), 249-259.

ACKNOWLEDGEMENTS

We would like to thank John and his parents for allowing us to present and publish this account. He has taught us a great deal. Acknowledgement is given to our colleagues at the Idylwild Center and University of Arizona who served as listeners. A special thanks goes to Cheryl Beeler and Felicia Simitoski, who helped tremendously in the development of listening tapes and in the presentation at the Conference.

Section III: Treatment

10

A Conceptual Holistic Approach To Dysarthria Treatment

Roxanne dePaul McNamara

INTRODUCTION

The assessment and treatment of dysarthria is viewed through various perspectives, Darley, Aronson, and Brown (1969a and b) offered a descriptive, perceptual approach, identifying 38 deviant speech dimensions in seven discrete neurological forms of acquired dysarthria. Each form of dysarthria reported had one or more patterns or clusters of deviant speech dimensions. This approach focuses on the differential diagnosis of dysarthric speech through the identification of deviant acoustic dimensions. Following this approach, treatment is designed to remediate the deviant perceptual symptomatology.

Overall measures of speech performance, particularly of speech intelligibility, have also been attempted as approaches to dysarthria intervention. Tikofsky and Tikofsky (1964) and, in subsequent papers, Tikofsky, Glattke, and Tikofsky (1966) and Tikofsky (1970) explored the possibility of developing quantifiable measures of speech intelligibility in dysarthria, such that measurement would facilitate a better estimate of the nature and extent of the dysarthric impairment.

More recently Yorkston and Beukelman (1978, 1980) and Beukelman and Yorkston (1979) have explored the quantification of overall communication function in dysarthria as sensitive measurements of subtle changes in speech performance. They have attempted to determine the relationship in information transfer; that is, successful communication and speech intelligibility (speaker to listener) as measured by single-word and paragraph transcription scores across a wide range of dysarthric speakers. Results of their work revealed a close relationship between transcription intelligibility scores and information transfer. Remediation is a communication-based approach with a focus on assessing baseline speech intelligibility and monitoring changes in speech intelligibility over time in treatment.

Netsell and Daniel (1979) described a physiologic component-by-component approach to dysarthria management. The selection and sequencing of intervention procedures is directly derived from the physiologic nature and severity of involvement in each component. Remediation focuses on the interrelationship of physiologic parameters and the application of biofeedback techniques in dysarthria treatment.

Is it possible, then, to integrate various perspectives on the assessment and treatment of dysarthria and to generate a holistic remediation approach ? Herein, using a case illustration, we will attempt to present a conceptual framework of an integrated approach to dysarthria treatment. This includes clinical procedures that reflect the equipment and ancillary personnel resources available in a typical rehabilitation setting.

Case History

M.G. was a 50-year-old female who suffered a CVA in May, 1980, with resultant severe left hemiplegia and brain stem involvement. She exhibited severe flaccid dysarthria characterized by severe intermittent aphonia and breathy phonation, hypernasality, and imprecise articulation. Speech was unintelligible. M.G. was nonambulatory and confined to a wheelchair. She also exhibited right eye blindness secondary to right choroidal artery hemorrhage in June, 1980. Before presenting M.G.'s assessment information in more depth, let us first review our basic evaluation procedures.

Diagnostic Evaluation

The following represents the procedural steps included in our routine diagnostic evaluation.

1. **Communication function** — Establishing an impression of communication funtion is the primary step in the diagnostic assessment.
This includes determining the client's pretreatment communication system. Judgments about the efficiency of the system are made. These include speech intelligibility measures, language abilities, and noting any sensory difficulties (for example, hearing or visual problems which may

interfere with communication). During the initial communication interaction, a self-defined or listener-defined perceptual gestalt of the client's speech acoustic symptomatology is established. A recently developed diagnostic tool, *Assessment of Intelligibility of Dysarthric Speech*, may be administered in order to quantify baseline speech intelligibility (Yorkston and Beukelman, 1981). At this time we attempt to decide whether an augmentative communication system would be needed as a temporary mode.

2. **PSM examination** — A peripheral speech mechanism examination is administered in order to carefully delineate the structural and functional adequacy of the oro-facial system. Specifically the degree of weakness, range of motion, and coordination of the oral facial musculature is assessed, along with measurements of nonspeech and speech (diadochokinesis) articulatory movements.

3. **Oral-articulatory inventory** — An oral-articulatory assessment is the administration of a standard articulation test. This assessment is useful for compiling a pretreatment inventory of oral-articulatory (placement) abilities within the context of a word. The test results provide information regarding baseline articulatory targets in treatment, particularly in severe dysarthria, when conversational speech is laboriously effected on a single word level. In addition, the static nature of this assessment affords the clinician an opportunity to identify obvious pretreatment compensatory strategies employed by the client.

4. **ENT evaluation** — A nasopharyngoscope is used by our cooperating otolaryngologist to evaluate velopharyngeal and laryngeal valving function during speech. The swallowing mechanism is also examined if dysphagia is present or suspected.

5. **Pulmonary function testing** — Pulmonary function testing is conducted upon request. However, air flow and pressure for speech purposes are not recorded due to the lack of appropriate instrumentation (Hardy, 1965; Borden and Harris, 1980). The Pulmonary Service will provide information regarding vegetative breathing.

Diagnostic Evaluation Results

A summary follows of the salient aspects of the diagnostic findings for M.G.

1. **Communication** — The combined effect of severely reduced oral-articulatory abilities, severely reduced vocal loudness, breathiness, intermittent aphonia, and severe nasal resonance resulted in non-functional oral communication. Augmentative communication is necessary. Speech intelligibility in actuality could not be rated. However, it was determined that M.G. had severely reduced vocal loudness with weak oral articulatory movement on single-word production. It was rated an equivalent of 6.5-7, using an equal appearing interval scale, with 0 equivalent to normal and 7 equivalent to unintelligible (Darley, Aronson, and Brown, 1969a; Netsell and Daniel, 1979). The severe nature of her dysarthria necessitated single-word ratings as opposed to conversational, paragraph, or sentence reading tasks.

2. **Oro-facial** — The oro-facial system revealed general weakness upon examination. Labial movements, particularly closure, were severely impaired due to the flaccidity of the lower lip. Tongue movements in all directions were weak; lingual-velar movements were visually absent. Overall strengthening, as well as improving oral-articulatory differentiation and active range of movement were indicated; therefore, the treatment implications here included devising a neurofacilitation program for flaccidity.

Results of the articulation test revealed severe oral-articulatory weakness, particularly with plosive and fricative production as expected with the velopharyngeal leak (See section 4). In addition to nasal emission, a compensatory lingual-dental (interdental) posture was noted for bilabial and lingual-alveolar placements.

3. **Laryngeal** — Nasopharyngoscopy revealed mild edema of the supraglottic larynx, and mild paresis of the left vocal cord during speech. Despite the presence of the paresis, the larynx was reported as within normal limits for phonation.

4. **Velopharyngeal** — The nasopharyngoscopic examination revealed an immobile velopharynx, with no visible movement of the posterior pharyngeal wall.

5. **Respiratory** — Pulmonary testing for vegetative breathing revealed a rapid tidal rate with fair tidal volume and markedly reduced vital capacity. The manometer measurements were poor, as expected, with considerable nasopharyngeal leak.

6. **Also** — Other significant findings included mild dysphagia for liquids, right eye blindness, and paralysis of the dominant left hand.

Treatment Selection

The presentation of treatment is based on the systematic selection and sequencing of multiple baselines as described by Netsell and Daniel (1979).

TABLE 10-1

AUGMENTATIVE COMMUNICATION PROFILE	
1. Speech:	nonfunctional
2. Language:	functional
3. Motor:	functional right hand (nondominant)
4. Sensory:	functional left eye functional hearing
5. Communication Needs:	communicate with family and unfamiliar (hospital) listeners

1. **Augmentative communication** — Table 10-1 lists the significant findings for augmentation. Recall that speech was nonfunctional in the presence of functional language. Motorically, she was able to utilize her right hand, since her dominant left hand was paralyzed. She exhibited functional vision in the left eye. Direct selection with the nondominant right hand served as the means for communicating in her augmentative system. Placement of any augmentative aid must be within her optimal field of vision due to the blindness. The type of augmentative system changed as M.G. progressed in speech treatment. Her options included: a) Writing as a viable alternative, although she felt it was too slow and illegible with her right hand; b) letterboard use, an inexpensive nonelectronic option (the letterboard was centered at body midline on her lapboard, with the letters facing the listener, and spelling was good, even with the letters upside down); c) the Canon Communicator, used temporarily at an early stage prior to speech remediation, since she was experiencing difficulty

maintaining nurses' attention to her letterboard messages (the Canon provided a written output, so she could prepare important messages in advance); d) the Speak n' Spell, with its synthesized speech output, also used at an early phase (she preferred using this device with her family); and, as speech remediation progressed and oral-articulatory and phonatory abilities improved, e) an amplifier was provided as augmentation to her speech output. The electronic aids were no longer viable, and she integrated amplified speech and letterboard use for communication. Speech and letterboard integration can be an effective and rapid communication system if listeners learn to predict words in context with two- and or three-letter cues by the user (Beukelman and Yorkston, 1977). In time, the amplifier was no longer required since vocal loudness became functional. Speech intelligibility continued to vary with listener familiarity; therefore, a letterboard became a permanent supplement for communication.

2. **Velopharyngeal** — The velopharyngeal component was considered first in speech treatment because, in addition to the perceived hypernasality, velopharyngeal incompetence might also account in part for M.G.'s severe reduction in perceived vocal loudness. Since abnormal coupling between the nasal and oral cavities significantly increases the damping characteristics of the vocal tract, it may have been sufficient to effect some reduction in perceived loudness. We hoped that the use of a palatal lift in this case would occlude the nasal port by holding the velum in contact with the posterior pharyngeal walls (Netsell and Daniel, 1979). We wanted to improve vocal loudness and decrease hypernasality with the overall result of improving speech intelligibility. Two problems existed in this plan, however. First M.G. was not willing to wear a prosthesis, even for a trial period, and, second, there was no prosthedontist on staff, necessitating an outside consultation. This could have been arranged providing the client was highly motivated and cooperative.

We decided to circumvent construction of a prosthesis early in the treatment plan due to the patient's unwillingness. Rather, we decided to continue to work to improve the oro-facial system, reasoning that improvement in oral-articulation would increase speech intelligibility. Further, we set up a vocal rehabilitation program that included clinical voice techniques, as well as biofeedback.

3. **Oro-facial** — A neurofacilitation program to reduce the flaccidity was implemented. A progressive intervention plan for improving articulation was developed, based on findings of the articulatory inventory gathered

from the formal articulation probe, as well as our impressions of co-articulatory breakdowns observed during conversational attempts. During early intervention, M.G. spoke one word at a time to effect conversation. Laborious single-word production provides little redundancy in the message and is a difficult listening task, particularly when the context is unknown. M.G., for example, was able to effect bilabial closure for production of an /m/ word in initial position when articulation was slow and deliberate. In a spontaneously generated context, /m/, words were produced with a lingual interdental placement. This was problematical for unfamiliar listeners. Although both productions were perceptually equivalent, her speech was not always decipherable acoustically, and visual cues were needed. Visual cues are significant message intelligibility aids when speech intelligibility is poor. Placement, in this example, illustrates how a listener's judgment can be miscued by the speaker when visual cues are crucial to understanding the message and do not conform to expectations.

4. **Laryngeal-Respiratory** — Measurement of laryngeal resistance through simultaneous recordings of air flow and pressure, as described by Smitheran and Hixon (1981), or individual recordings of air flow and air pressure, as described by Netsell and Daniel (1979), would have been applicable to this case, both diagnostically and therapeutically, for biofeedback. However, such equipment was not accessible. We speculated that the laryngeal dysfunction was apparently related to faulty valving due to the paresis, resulting in an inadequate build-up of subglottal air pressure. That is, subglottal air pressure was probably less than the clinical rule of thumb value, or 5cm H_2O maintained for five seconds (Netsell and Hixon, 1978). The breathiness may have been indicative of inefficient modulation of air; that is, laryngeal airway resistance during vowel phonation was probably inadequate (as discussed by Smitheran and Hixon, 1981), resulting in excessive air flow or air wastage through the system.

Another perspective on the problem, however, given the pulmonary test results, was that M.G. had difficulty generating and/or maintaining adequate air flow. Nasal coupling compounded the problem by creating a larger area for the dissipating air to flow through. Hence, supraglottal pressure for oral-articulatory gestures was significantly reduced. This required her to engage in greater expiratory efforts for all speech attempts, in order to compensate for the velopharyngeal leak.

Treatment was initiated with traditional hypertonic exercises in an attempt to strengthen the paretic vocal cord by improving laryngeal resistance. Minimal change was noted perceptually. Use of the Kay Visi-

Pitch (Kay Elemetrics, 1979) with visual feedback, appeared to improve vocal loudness. At the time, our clinic did not have a permanent recording system to gather data from the Visi-Pitch.

Frustrated by the poor results and the lack of objective measurement, we developed, with consultation from a colleague,[1] a simple biofeedback paradigm, which may have a range of potential applications in dysarthria treatment. The instrumentation included a sequential panel of lights, a clock, and a microphone.

Phase one in biofeedback was to facilitate voice onset of an isolated vowel. Vocal intensity was measured on a relative scale from 0 to 10. Ten was most sensitive and could be activated by a whisper, whereas 0 required considerable effort. A successful trial was rewarded by activation of the light panel.

Phase two was initiated when M.G. was able to phonate consistently on command. Increased duration of phonation was the next goal. Voice onset continued to activate the light panel; however, the clock rotated upon initiation of voice and recorded the length of phonation. Intensity was again recorded, relatively, from 0-10. M.G. worked to keep the clock moving. Performance on this task was variable.

This method recorded changes in the loudness and durational aspects of sustained vowel phonation; that is, it was a direct measure of a particular outcome. The technique offered a way to quantify performance, and resulted in objective, as well as perceptual, improvements in loudness.

We attempted to account for one phonatory element by measuring habitual pitch, using the Kay Visi-Pitch. Her average habitual pitch range was 152-163Hz. Measurement of sustained vowel phonations on good biofeedback performance days, when loudness was audible and duration improved, indicated an average fundamental frequency of 183Hz. M.G. was compensating for reduced vocal loudness by raising pitch, and probably engaging in greater expiratory effort (Isshiki and von Leden, 1964). Improvements in the durational aspects of speech were less successful, apparently due to the combined effect of inefficient laryngeal resistance and air wastage. The biofeedback treatment, in conjunction with oral-articulatory management, resulted in increasing vocal loudness, with a mild decrease in the perception of hypernasality during conversational attempts.

CONCLUSIONS

Table 10-2 illustrates the multiple treatment baselines presented hypothetically, but in sequence (Netsell and Daniel, 1979).

TABLE 10-2

SYSTEM	WEEKS OF TREATMENT												
	0	1	2	3	4	5	6	7	8	9	10	11	12
1. Augmentative	XXXXXXXXXXXXXXXXXXXXXXXXXXXXXXX
2. Oro-facial	XXXXXXXXXXXXXXXXXXXXXXXXXXXX
3. Laryngeal	XXXXXXXXXXXXXXXXXXXXXXXXX
4. Respiratory	XXXXXXXXXXXXXXXXXXXXXXXXX
5. Velopharyngeal*	XXX...............................

under consideration

Augmentation continued throughout intervention, although the nature of the augmentative system was altered throughout the course of treatment. M.G. will always need a letterboard for unfamiliar listeners.

Oro-facial intervention was initiated early with an oro-neuro-facilitation program, which was decreased during treatment. Intervention in oral articulation was a primary focus, with the premise that improved oral-articulatory skill would increase speech intelligibility.

The laryngeal and respiratory systems were approached through vocal rehabilitation and biofeedback. Intermittent aphonia and reduced vocal loudness remained as predominant symptoms in M.G.'s speech pattern.

Velopharyngeal management had always been under consideration. However, the decision was to maximize the other system components before attempting to proceed with the construction of a palatal lift and convincing the patient she must wear the prosthesis for a trial period.

The overall effect of this intervention was significant improvement in speech intelligibility. Coversational speech was typically paced in short, deliberate phrases. Reduced vocal loudness, breathiness with intermittent aphonia, and hypernasality continued to characterize her dysarthric speech. However, M.G. was able to depend on speech as a primary mode of communication, integrating letterboard use only when message intelligibility was undecipherable by a listener.

This case illustration demonstrates a holistic approach to the treatment of dysarthria. Clearly, the severity and complexity of M.G.'s communication impairment necessitated an integrated approach to treatment. We feel that systematic selection and sequencing of intervention procedures provides the clinician with a logical and creative problem-solving approach in which objective measurement techniques are easily applied. Specifically, the variety of techniques employed provides the client with a network of optimal strategies that may be used in various communicative situations.

NOTE

[1]Dr. Bernard S. Brucker, formerly Senior Pathologist at Goldwater Memorial Hospital, is presently Director of the Psychology Service in the Department of Orthopaedics and Rehabilitation at the University of Miami Medical Center and School of Medicine.

REFERENCES

Beukelman, D., & Yorkston, K. A communication system for the severely dysarthric speaker with an intact language system. *Journal of Speech and Hearing Disorders*, 1977, *42*, 265-270.

Beukelman, D., & Yorkston, K. The relationship between information transfer and speech intelligibility of dysarthric speakers. *Journal of Communicative Disorders*, 1979, *12*, 189-196.

Borden, G., & Harris, K. *Speech science primer*. Baltimore: Williams & Wilkins, 1980.

Darley, F., Aronson, A., & Brown, J. Differential diagnostic patterns of dysarthria. *Journal of Speech and Hearing Research*, 1969, *12*, 246-269. (a)

Darley, F., Aronson, A., & Brown, J. Clusters of deviant speech dimensions in the dysarthrias. *Journal of Speech and Hearing Research*, 1969, *12*, 462-496. (b)

Hardy, J. Air flow and air pressure studies. *ASHA Reports*, 1965, *1*, 141-152.

Isshiki, N., & von Leden, H. Hoarseness: Aerodynamics studies. *Archives of Otolaryngology*, 1964, *80*, 206-213.

Kay Elemetrics Corporation. "Visi-Pitch application notes — Diagnosis and treatment of voice disorders." 1979.

Netsell, R., & Daniel, B. Dysarthria in adults: Physiologic approach to rehabilitation. *Archives of Physical Medicine and Rehabilitation*, 1979, *60*, 502-508.

Netsell, R., & Hixon, T. Noninvasive method for clinically estimating subglottal air pressure. *Journal of Speech and Hearing Disorders*, 1978, *43*, 326-330.

Smitheran, J., & Hixon, T. A clinical method for estimating laryngeal airway resistance during vowel production. *Journal of Speech and Hearing Disorders*, 1981, *46*, 138-146.

Tikofsky, R. A revised list for the estimation of dysarthric single word intelligibility. *Journal of Speech and Hearing Research*, 1970, *13*, 59-64.

Tikofsky, R., Glattke, T., & Tikofsky, R. Listener confusions in response to dysarthric speech. *Folia Phoniatria*, 1966, *18*, 280-292.

Tikofsky, R., & Tikofsky, R. Intelligibility measures of dsyarthric speech. *Journal of Speech and Hearing Research*, 1964, *7*, 325-333.

Yorkston, K., & Beukelman, D. A comparison of techniques for measuring intelligibility of dysarthric speech. *Journal of Communicative Disorders*, 1978, *11*, 499-512.

Yorkston, K., & Beukelman, D. A clinical-judged technique for quantifying dysarthric speech based on single-word intelligibility. *Journal of Communicative Disorders*, 1980, *13*, 15-31.

Yorkston, K., & Beukelman, D. *Assessment of intelligibility of dysarthric speech*, Tigard, OR: C.C. Publications, 1981.

11

Environmental Education: The Universal Management Approach for Adults with Dysarthria

William R. Berry
Sara B. Sanders

INTRODUCTION

It is a commonly accepted notion that treatment of dysarthric symptoms seldom leads to normal speech. As speech pathologists, we generally hope to reduce the severity of the symptoms, or to alter speech behaviors in some way to produce an increase in speech intelligibility. We may be confronted with a degenerative condition like amyotrophic lateral sclerosis (ALS) or multiple sclerosis (MS), where the patient's speech will ultimately get worse, no matter who the clinician is or what is done. The ethics of continued treatment may even become questionable when a neurologist refers a patient with degenerative disease to a speech pathologist. There are some who question the efficacy of referring any adult with dysarthria to a speech clinician, regardless of neurologic prognosis. Physicians often question the cost effectiveness of behavioral symptomatic treatment involving patients with neurologic disease. When this happens, the physician is taking a "triage" approach to referral, given what s(he) knows about the patient, the neurological disorder, the course of disease, the prognosis for recovery, and his/her knowledge of speech pathology.

If the primary care physician, generally a neurologist in the case of dysarthric adults, was aware that speech pathology had more to offer his patients than merely motoric retraining (i.e., therapy) in treating dysarthria, there would be less hesitation in referring patients. *Environmental Education* is a total rehabilitation approach that could help to break down some of the negative attitudes that often impede referral. and we feel that it is almost universal in the overall treatment model. Consider one such model of treatment involving dysarthric adults.

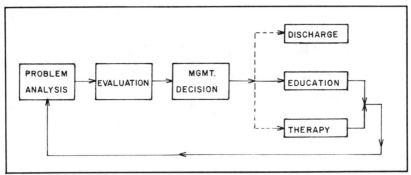

FIGURE 11-1
Schematic flow chart illustrating stages in clinical management of dysarthric patients.

Solid lines in Figure 11-1 indicate mandatory action by the speech clinician, beginning with an analysis of the communicative problems reported by the patient, as well as other significant informants in the dysarthric's communicative environment. This "problem analysis" is followed by a comprehensive evaluation of the patient's speech, which leads to clinical management decisions. There are three general decisions that can be made after the assessment. First, treatment may not be indicated, hence the contingency of discharge, and the treatment flow chart ends at that point. If treatment is pursued, the model postulates one mandatory course of management and another contingent upon a number of variables.

The latter involves some type of therapeutic intervention to improve or alter speech behaviors. This may be undertaken by the speech clinician or by someone else on the treatment team, such as a prosthodontist, a neurologist, a physical therapist, or a surgeon. The "therapy" might be behavioral, prosthetic equipment, drugs, diet education, exercise, surgery, or a combination of these, with the goal of improved intelligibility for the patient. There are times, however, when individual therapy is not pursued. The reasons may be medical/neurological, psychosocial, practical, or personal. Nevertheless, in almost every instance, an adult with dysarthria can benefit from *Environmental Education*, the third and mandatory management decision following the evaluation.

Environmental Education is the process of providing pertinent information that, if applied by the dysarthric adult and those in the environment, will facilitate an improvement in the patient's intelligibility. Even if the patient resists teaching, verbal communication with the dysarthric can be improved if the significant persons who interact with the patient learn more about their loved one's communication.

APPLICATION

Environmental Education is certainly not a new approach to communication. Quite simply, it is the application of teaching principles involved in aural rehabilitation as they apply to the other aspects of verbal communication (i.e., the speech-impaired patient). It is important to emphasize that, if any speech rehabilitation is undertaken, the environmental educational process should be an important part of that protocol. It may even be the exclusive emphasis of treatment, especially when the prognosis for improved intelligibility is negative. All too often, we have observed patients who were sent home to cope with the admonition that "therapy simply won't help your speech."

In our treatment model, individual therapy may or may not be appropriate. However, *Environmental Education* can be implemented with almost every dysarthric adult. All that is necessary is a patient, or someone in the environment, who is willing to learn and who is capable of acting on the principles that are taught. Note that we may achieve progress in verbal interaction through *Environmental Education* using an indirect learning process. This will become more obvious as the principles are explained.

The roots of *Environmental Education* are found in aural rehabilitation. A hearing-impaired individual, especially one who has become so later in life, must learn a set of interaction "rules" that, if ignored, lead to great difficulties when communicating verbally with others. These admonitions are well-established. Here are a few.

1. Avoid noisy, dark places. If encountered, move away from the noise when listening, or into an area of increased lighting.

2. The telephone may provide a major obstacle to communication unless special amplification can be of help.

3. Move closer to the person who is speaking; a distance of 3-6 feet with a full face view maximizes intelligibility.

4. A hearing aid will not help if it is in a drawer at home.

5. Encourage friends to speak more slowly; don't be afraid to admit you have a hearing problem.

Attempts to teach these points have always been part of aural rehab. However, the emphasis for many years was on lip reading or speech reading. More recently, rehabilitation audiologists have begun to teach a wider scope of universal communication skills with an emphasis on what the hearing impaired individual *can do* rather than on the handicap in the communication process. It is obvious that a program such as that had application for any speech impaired-adult who was having difficulty being understood. At least one important factor became apparent to us: When adults, who have been reasonably effective communicators, lose hearing or speaking skills, some find it difficult to utilize and develop residual communication skills. The objective of *Environmental Education* is to promote the development of these communication skills. If the principles of aural rehab education are applied by the dysarthric adult, not only verbal communication but his/her life style may be enhanced.

The essence of our discussion is a rather simple model of verbal information transfer that can help the clinician remember a number of variables that should be incorporated into the *Environmental Education* process.

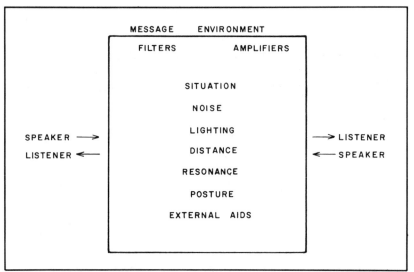

FIGURE 11-2
A schematic illustration of variables in the message environment that will affect the intelligibility of verbal communication.

In figure 11-2 we conceptualize a message environment through which each speaker/listener must send or receive verbal messages. With the dysarthric adult, we will assume that the listener, whoever that might be, is a normal hearing individual with normal auditory comprehension. If this is not the case, it is obvious that the clinician must apply aural rehab principles and work actively with this listener in the treatment process, especially if the listener is a spouse or family member of the dysarthric individual.

Assuming a normal listener, however, as well as normal listening skills on the part of the dysarthric, we can further develop our model. In the message environment, our dysarthric and his listener(s) will confront a number of variables that may be compared to filters and/or amplifiers. Depending upon the presence and character of the variables listed in the model, the verbal message will be altered in its intelligibility. It follows, therefore, that an increased awareness of these factors, and selective control of them, could have a positive effect upon the reliability of verbal message transfer. Following is a description of the variables and their effects on the patient and listener.

Situation

Situation refers to the moment in time that the message occurs, and all the learned expectations surrounding the message. It is the where, when, who, why, and the what of the message. All of us have been in situations where we only understood part of what was said, but were able to "fill in" the rest due to the predictability of the message content for the situation. The converse is also true. We might try to anticipate what a person is going to say, but the speaker has something else in mind and communicates an unpredictable message. The speech-impaired patient and his/her listeners should be taught to use the situation as a tool, learning to anticipate what might be said in given situations, actually thinking about possible messages ahead of time, and learning to control context or situational cues as much as possible. For example, when a dysarthric speaker is talking on the phone and wants to change topics, s(he) should learn to set the context for a listener. A preparatory carrier phrase like ". . .I want to talk about — (pause) — *Thanksgiving dinner* (pronounced slowly/distinctly). . ." could be used to allow the listener to change his preparatory listening set. This strategy, once learned by the dysarthric would make telephoning or other problem situations less tedious, frustrating, and/or embarrassing. Listeners must also learn to anticipate a message, especially with the severe dysarthric; and they should also be alert while listening, asking appropriate, context questions when necessary.

Noise

Noise is a common nemesis to intelligibility, even with normal speakers/listeners. The most common strategy that we all use to overcome noise is to speak louder. This may work occasionally for speakers with normal neuromuscular speech mechanisms. However, when one who suffers from severe ataxia, hyperkinesia, or spasticity uses this pattern, it proves counterproductive to intelligibility because the patient's speech control mechanisms are not operating properly. The extra effort tends to "overdrive" the available speech mechanism and create hyperdistorted speech, which is even more difficult for the listener to understand. The dysarthric and the listener must be taught other, more productive strategies, such as the following:

1. If the noise is variable, turn it down. Put the patient in control of TV or radio loudness. Turning a TV down signals to all listeners that the dysarthric wants to speak, diverting visual attention to the patient.

2. If the noise cannot be controlled, the patient may move away from the noise source to a quieter area (or moving closer to one another might help).

3. Visual attention is extremely important! The speaker must learn (and it cannot be assumed that he will learn this automatically) to get direct eye-contact with the listener. The use of the listener's name, or a touch of the arm, will increase intelligibility of the message to follow.

4. The dysarthric must not use louder speech, but, rather, move closer to the listener, speaking slowly and as precisely as possible to facilitate reliable message transfer. Using a slower rate of speech with judicious pauses must also be learned in therapy by many dysarthric patients, and then applied in noisy situations. This is especially true for patients with ataxic or hypokinetic dysarthria. In these instances, symptomatic speech therapy and environmental education compliment each other.

You will probably recognize that the suggestions can also be applied with hearing-impaired individuals who confront a noisy environment. The remaining variables in our model also apply to both populations of communicatively impaired adults, or with children for that matter. The only difference between age groups would be in the amount and application of learned or over-learned speech/language habits that are applied to these speaking situations.

Lighting

Lighting is an important consideration if a listener needs speech reading cues to understand a dysarthric patient. Turning the lights off or down in a TV room may enhance visualization of the tube, but makes it more difficult for the dysarthric to be understood. Candlelight dinners may be romantic but may also promote frustration due to the reduced intelligibility. Teach your patient to sit in a well-lighted area, especially in a restaurant or night club. Remember, these situations may also be complicated by high ambient noise, which increases the need for lighting.

Distance

Distance, which has already been mentioned in the context of ambient noise, is another feature of environmental control. ANSI standards for rating noise with respect to speech interference[1] indicate that in communication involving normal-speaking adults, a speaker talking at a normal intensity level should not be farther than four feet from the listener out-of-doors, if the interfering noise level is 55 dB. This is a relatively low level of ambient noise. Indoors, one must be closer because of the resonant properties of most rooms, which reflect the interfering noise. These data tell us that we must make our dysarthric speakers more aware of the distance factor because their tendency will be to speak louder, rather than to reduce the distance from speaker to listener.

Resonance

Resonance is an extremely complex variable that is not fully understood. These recommendations to your patient may help:

1. If expense does not prohibit, noise dampening by carpeting, selective wall or furniture covering (as thick and porous as possible), and/or heavy draperies will allow the patient to speak at lower loudness levels to facilitate accurate intelligibility.

2. The patient and listeners should be aware of the effects of hard walls, so that when they enter such an environment they can take steps to improve message transfer, such as moving closer to each other or away from a noise, attending more closely to visual cues, using more gestures, or simply waiting to communicate until the environment is quieter or the participants are in a different place.

Posture

Posture refers to the physical placement of the speaker and the listener/observer in the message environment. Whenever possible in any group conversation, a dysarthric should be situated so that all listeners in the group can have a full-face view of the speaker. At dinner, he should be seated at the head of the table, not on the side where some listeners might have only a profile view. A dysarthric in a wheelchair should attempt to seat himself facing a listener at every opportunity, which maximizes attention to the speaker, minimizes distance, and promotes visualization.

External Aids

External Aids can be used to facilitate intelligibility. These aids can be used by the speaker, the listener, or both, depending upon the abilities of the message sender or the receiver. For example, an adult with mild dysarthria may have a parent with severe hearing loss, probably high frequency presbycusis, and a hearing aid or some other amplification device may be indicated. Selective amplification for the dysarthric may be necessary. A patient suffering from unilateral vocal fold paralysis will likely have a breathy voice, reduced in loudness. Speaking loudly (in a hyper-whisper, or a loud, harsh, breathy voice) may lead to rapid vocal fatigue, inefficient use of the air stream, and vocal abuse. A larger, more permanent amplification system should be used if the person must use his low intensity voice on a regular basis. A portable system should be encouraged for more informal situations. Telephone amplifiers are available to boost the signal of the sender as well as the receiver.

Other external aids are available—albeit with some significant expense— for the severely dysarthric or anarthric adult. Microelectronics and computers now provide severely-involved dysarthrics with alternative modes of communication. Other aids such as communication boards are used effectively by many patients, especially those in limited/restricted environments (e.g., bedfast patients) to communicate their basic needs. Communication board systems are limited to more concrete communication needs, but can be very helpful in certain situations, especially when the patient is not capable of operating a more advanced microelectronics device.

SUMMARY

These are the major variables that must be systematically considered when *Environmental Education* is used in the management of the adult with dysarthria. These variables can be used as a checklist in assessing a patient's verbal effectiveness in specific environmental situations. A number of factors should be considered when using *Environmental Education.*

1. Do not assume that patients/listeners are aware of the variables affecting intelligibility, or that they will learn to control them effectively on their own.

2. An evaluation of environmental communication skills, as well as speech behaviors, is encouraged.

3. An aggressive attempt should be made to involve the significant others who serve as listeners in the patient's environment, especially when the dysarthric is more severely involved or only marginally cooperative.

4. Follow-up information should be gathered concerning the patients' and/or listeners' understanding of what is being taught. Every subjective report of communicative success received by the patient, listeners, or others should be entered in progress reports.

Of these four factors, two indicate that systematic assessment and data gathering are important when *Environmental Education* is part of your clinical management program. This is also implied by the overall treatment model in Figure 11-1. In an attempt to enhance our basic evaluation of the adult dysarthric and provide standardized information about the patient in his communicative environment, we are developing a Situation Intelligibility Survey (SIS) which can be found in Appendix A. The SIS is administered to the patient and/or key informants (i.e., generally, primary listeners in the patient's environment). A verbal question-answer format is used, in which the patient or the informant is asked general, but leading, questions, such as "Does anybody have trouble understanding what you say (or he says)?" or, "Where do you have the most trouble?" Questions can, of course, be more specific if necessary: for example, "Do people have trouble understanding you on the phone? . . . all the time or part of the time?" This question allows the clinician to score one of the items on the SIS, using the scale provided. Twenty situations are used for the initial survey and there is space for up to five others which can be added by the clinician based upon the interview. The total possible score on the SIS would be the number of total situations multiplied by a factor of two. A percentage score can then be derived which roughly reflects the perceived intelligibility on any given date. Obviously, the SIS results can also help the clinician to isolate situations where the patient or others in the environment might need instruction. SIS, having been administered to the patient and other informants, can also serve to gather information and compare various perceptions of the patient's intelligibility problems. This evaluation protocol is in its infancy; however, we think that this, or some form of survey, can provide a systematic and somewhat standardized method for assessing the patient's environmental communication before, during, and after treatment. Ideally, it will also provide information about the efficacy of an *Environmental Education* program.

Going back to our treatment model (Figure 11-1), once the patient and others have presented the problems, the patient has been evaluated (including SIS or some equivalent), and a decision has been made to pursue some form of treatment, we are postulating that *Environmental Education* should be implemented. The only exception to this would be a refusal to cooperate by the patient and the fact that *no one* in the patient's environment could be contacted, or was interested in the program. Generally, the patient is willing and/or someone can be located who will cooperate. Individual or group instructional sessions can be used, dictated by practical considerations and caseload scheduling priorities. We have found it helpful to use handouts like the one in Appendix B to facilitate instruction. Besides more traditional didactics, role-playing sessions are of obvious value. Telephone treatment can be of special value, especially when talking on the telephone presents a particular problem, or when travel for this instruction is difficult. Though we have not actively pursued the program of communication workshops for a number of families of dysarthric speakers, we feel this would be valuable. Just as those that have been used to educate hearing aid users and their families, these workshops would allow our patients to focus on the positive aspects of communication, rather than allowing them to dwell upon the individual's disability.

The *Environmental Education* program—either singularly as the treatment of choice, or in conjunction with some specific mode of therapy to improve speech symptoms—should be pursued until the clinician is assured that learning has been maximized, or that no learning has taken place given a reasonable attempt. This is measured by methods such as the SIS, subjective reports from the patient or significant others, oral examination relative to the points covered in the program, and/or the clinician's impression. The process generally takes about 3-6 one-hour sessions.

To further illustrate the program: Mr. R., a moderate spastic/ataxic dysarthric who was approximately 23-30% intelligible, began a combined treatment approach to include environmental education and symptomatic therapy. To improve or alter speech behaviors, a number of goals were pursued: (1) reduction of laryngeal tension by relaxation exercises, emphasizing an easy onset of phonation and decreasing phonatory effort; (2) reducing rate of speech by increasing vowel duration and pause time; (3) improving articulatory precision by stressing initial consonant production and syllabilizing words of increased length, and specific drills to improve diadochokinetic skills; and (4) increasing the amount of inflection or prosody in his speech by altering duration and loudness.

These behavioral alterations by themselves were not adequate to eliminate Mr. R's intelligibility problems, without also attempting to make him more aware of his environment and the interaction with his listeners. Adhering to the model in Figure 11-2, several variables in the message environment needed to be controlled by the patient. Mr. R. was taught to increase his control of the communicative situation by establishing the topic to be discussed before the specific interaction began. If he were the sender of a message, he began his verbal interaction by stating his intent to discuss a particular context.

One of the most important variables to be controlled was noise in the environment. Our patient was in the habit of trying to talk above ambient noise before we began our therapy protocol. Mr. R. learned to avoid talking in extremely noisy environments, to turn the noise down when possible, and to use optimal positioning in less noisy environments — such as moving away from the source of the noise or moving closer to the listener. At all times, the patient made sure that he was well-visualized either by strategic posturing or by good lighting. He became quite adept at asking his listeners periodically if they understood what he had said. His perception of the listener's body language and/or facial expressions was quite well-developed after approximately six weeks of treatment.

Follow-up evaluation at the end of six weeks indicated significant improvement in Mr. R.'s communication skills. Overall phonation became more periodic, rate of speech was 79% slower, consonant identification on acoustical tracings increased from 64% to 100%, electroglottography revealed increased periodicity during voluntary alteration of pitch and loudness, and intelligibility increased from 27% to 82%. Most important however, was the patient's report that, except for strangers, almost everyone with whom he communicated indicated they understood him much better than they had previously. In fact, he enjoys playing a tape recording for his friends of his speech before he began this therapy protocol. He always laughs and says, "If you can understand that, then you're a lot better than me; I can't understand one word, and I'm doing the talking."

Mr. R., though highly motivated and intelligent, is not an isolated case. He and those in his environment who learned more about the process of communication and applied many of the positive principles/suggestions outlined herein, have definitely benefited from our *Environmental Education* program. Many others have, as well. In fact, only those who refuse to cooperate, or cannot learn, do not benefit, which is an extremely small number. We hope that clinicians will see the applications of *Environmental Education* and the simplicity with which this program can be implemented for the adult with any type, or severity, of dysarthria.

APPENDIX A

Situational Intelligibility Survey (SIS)

People have trouble understanding me, him/her: SCORE

    1. everywhere   _____
    2. in noisy places   _____
    3. in dark places   _____
    4. when strangers are the listeners   _____
    5. in group conversation   _____
    6. when watching TV/listening to radio   _____
    7. in stores   _____
    8. in restaurants/night spots   _____
    9. on the phone   _____
   10. while in a car   _____
   11. when I am sitting   _____
   12. when I am walking   _____
   13. when I am tired   _____
   14. when I am emotional   _____
   15. in the morning   _____
   16. in the afternoon   _____
   17. at night   _____
   18. at a distance of 5 ft. (when quiet)   _____
   19. at a distance of 10 ft. (when quiet)   _____
   20. at a distance of 15 ft. (when quiet)   _____
   21.   _____
   22.   _____
   23.   _____
   24.   _____
   25.   _____

Scoring Scale: All the time Occasionally Never
                0   1   2

Informant/Patient : _____ Total Score = _____

Date   : _____ Total Possible= _____

Clinician   : _____ % Score   = _____ %

APPENDIX B

Suggestions to Improve your Communication

*In noisy situations:

- Do not speak louder to overcome the noise.

- Turn the noise off or move away from it, if possible.

- Get eye contact while speaking.

- Anticipate; use situational cues.

- Talk slower; rephrase when repeating, when necessary.

- Pay attention to body language and gestures.

*On the Telephone:

- Sit upright, hold receiver near mouth.

- Speak more slowly than usual.

- Announce any subject (or change) with key words.

- Use amplifier if necessary.

*At Dinner or in Groups:

- Make sure all see speaker's face (front view).

- Use key word cues to announce change of subject.

- Maintain eye contact with group.

- Do not try to speak more loudly because of group.

- Avoid dark or noisy areas for group conversations.

*When Asked to Repeat:

- Do NOT repeat at louder level.

- Rephrase and speak more slowly.

- Use gestures and other cues.

- Move closer to listener if possible.

*When Watching TV/Listening to Radio:

- Patient in control of audio loudness (remote, if possible).

- Cue with loudness for attention; wait for eye contact.

NOTES

[1]Acoustical Society of America, *American National Standard for Rating Noise with Respect to Speech Interference,* 1977, American Institute of Physics, New York, 1-4.

12

Treatment of a Four-Year-Old With a Palatal Lift Prosthesis

Ann L. Shaughnessy
Ronald Netsell
James Farrage

INTRODUCTION

In this detailed case study, several diagnostic and treatment procedures are drawn from our experiences with adult dysarthrics (Netsell and Rosenbek, in preparation), and applied to an unintelligible four-year-old boy. Even though the etiology of his speech disorder is unclear, these clinical procedures were successful where others had failed. We consider his case germane because these principles and procedures are useful with children variously labeled as developmentally delayed, dysarthric, and/or dyspraxic.

SUBJECT DESCRIPTION

History

Kevin was brought to the Boys Town Institute at age three by his parents. They reported concern for his delayed speech development and lack of interest in talking.

Prenatal history indicated a normal pregnancy with Actifed taken for hay fever. Labor and delivery were unremarkable and birth weight was seven pounds, six ounces. His parents were in their mid-twenties at the time of his birth. He has one sister, 16 months older, who is normal.

A heart murmur was identified at birth; subsequently Tetralogy of Fallot was diagnosed. Corrective heart surgery was performed at age 27 months. Kevin also suffered frequent colds, croup, and pneumonia, usually accompanied by high fever.

His mother stated that prior to surgery, Kevin had poor respiratory function and breath support for all activities. He was not walking and would often squat, apparently to improve respiration. This observation suggests the possibility of reduced subglottal air pressure for vocalization. He engaged in limited babbling, cooing, and sound making in early childhood. A loss of liquid through the nose had occurred since infancy and still was seen infrequently at age three. No other problems with feeding function were reported.

Diagnostic Findings

A multidisciplinary evaluation was completed. Initial diagnostic findings indicated average nonverbal intelligence, normal receptive

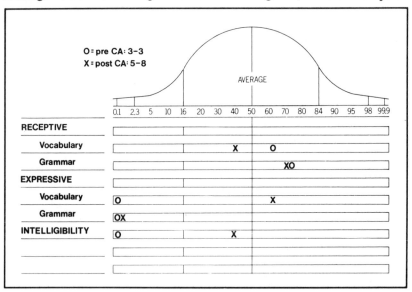

FIGURE 12-1

A profile of results of speech/language testing (pre- and post-therapy)

*Plotted on a normal curve relative to chronological age. The 50th percentile for intelligibility is considered 100 percent intelligible for an average child. 0=pre-therapy score and X=post-therapy score

language, normal auditory memory and visual skills, average adaptive behavior skills, adequate vegetative movements of the oral musculature, and manual motor skills in the borderline range. Kevin demonstrated a severe expressive language delay of approximately two years, gross motor and personal-social skills below normal, and poor stimulability for correction of speech errors. Speech output was characterized by undifferentiated vowels, guttural sounds, and airflow directed nasally (See Figure 12-1).

Additional medical findings failed to reveal a genetic syndrome, and there was no evidence of short or cleft palate. Brainstem auditory-evoked responses were normal. Results of videofluoroscopy were indeterminate but "abnormal palatal motion" was suspected. Adenoidal tissue, although slightly reduced, was considered within normal limits. Neurologic findings were inconclusive regarding the cause of the velopharyngeal incompetence and speech delay.

Following the evaluation, Kevin was placed in a preschool language group program. The objectives were to develop personal-social skills, increase motivation for use of verbal language, and provide opportunities to attempt new gross motor skills through interactions with other children. The program was geared to provide continuous language stimulation, and small group language and articulation therapy.

INTERVENTION: PHASE I

CA: 3-3 to 4-0

The preschool language group program is considered Phase I of Kevin's remediation program. The group was based on a cognitively oriented curriculum. Goals were established to develop linguistic structure, receptive and expressive vocabulary, and a variety of other language functions. Procedures for language therapy will not be detailed here. It is noteworthy that approximately eighty percent of the program each day was alloted to language and twenty percent to articulation. Articulation goals in Phase I included: (1) establishing adequate vowel productions, (2) stimulation of nasals and vowels in syllable combinations, (3) establishing oral airflow with imitation of /h/, (4) shaping production of oral plosives from lip smacking and tongue clicks, (5) probing ability to imitate visible, non-nasal consonants, (6) establishing oral airflow in nonspeech activities, and (7) stimulating /s/ productions with the nose plugged.

Progress during Phase I, a period of approximately ten months, was most notable in the production of vowels. Use of /n/ in single syllable word approximations (i.e., *no, in, on*) was reported. Kevin could produce

/h/ in isolation but not in longer sequences. His ability to direct airflow orally reported by improved for nonspeech tasks but nasal airflow was always present as well. Attempts to establish productions of oral consonants were unsuccessful.

Improvement in functioning of the front tongue was suggested by spontaneous use of /l/ in a word, *little*. Also, it was reported that /p, b/ were perceived infrequently when Kevin was not thinking about what he was trying to say.

One therapy procedure was to plug the nose and stimulate for /s/ production. The use of nose plugs to block nasal airflow and provide oral pressure for valving is a technique which has been used successfully as a diagnostic tool with dysarthric adults. The blocking of nasal airflow at the nares may provide the dysarthric with the necessary oral pressure to demonstrate a marked improvement in articulation (see Jamieson, Matsko, Snyder, and Riegger, 1981).

The use of nose plugs in Kevin's case was counterproductive. He had no previous experience producing oral consonants and did not appear to know how to valve the oral air. With the plugs in place, he imitated the /s/ stimulus by attempting to force air through his nose without correct lingual valving. Also, the oral fricative appeared to be a strong, salient feature, as he tended to produce it prior to all speech attempts. Thus, this case suggests plugging the nares may not be appropriate in an individual without past experience of articulatory oral airflow.

A majority of the articulation goals in this phase were directed toward establishing oral productions and improving velopharyngeal function. Results were poor. Assessment following Phase I indicated Kevin had maintained adequate vowel productions, use of /n/ in the word *no*, and /m/ in short, common words.

Based on Kevin's performance in Phase I, he was given the diagnosis of developmental apraxia of speech. The following characteristics gleaned from the literature were applied: (1) adequate strength and movement of his motor speech components for vegetative and nonspeech movements, (2) unintelligible speech due to a severely limited repertoire consisting of vowel productions and limited production of /m/ and /n/, (3) inconsistent errors on vowel productions, (4) evidence of oral-nonverbal apraxia, (5) groping for placement of articulators, (6) poor progress in therapy, (7) difficulty imitating sequences of sound, (8) no evidence of aphasia or receptive language deficits, and (9) poor response to stimulation.

As a result of this diagnosis, Kevin was referred to one of us (Shaughnessy) for intensive, individual therapy, primarily because of her experience in treating adults with apraxia of speech.

Kevin remained in the preschool and participated in the language activities. Shortly after he began therapy (Phase II), a program to teach him sign language was initiated. The clinicians in the language group considered his prognosis so poor as to warrant a manual communication system.

INTERVENTION: PHASE II.

CA: 4-0 to 4-8

Phase II of Kevin's remediation, approximately eight months in duration, refers to the period of intensive therapy prior to the fitting of the palatal lift. An initial step was to re-examine the label of developmental apraxia. We (Shaughnessy and Netsell) questioned the presence of a motor programming deficit that was inferred from his inability to produce single or sequenced speech sounds that were not within his physiologic capabilities. We considered it appropriate to design production and sequencing tasks within his physiologic capacity to determine speech motor programming potential. In essence, this constituted sequences employing nasal consonants and vowels. This will be discussed below.

Early in Phase II, we suspected that the presence of velopharyngeal incompetence was a major contributing factor to Kevin's reduced intelligibility and limited articulation. Although the cause of the velopharyngeal problem was not known and we lacked evidence that alleviating it would improve his articulation, we determined that it was necessary to manage this aspect of Kevin's speech disorder. Kevin's history suggested that velopharyngeal incompetence had been present since infancy and therapy in Phase I failed to yield a significant increase in velopharyngeal function. We felt, therefore, that prosthetic management with a palatal lift was warranted. The advantages of a palatal lift over surgical repair include the (1) ability to modify lift size to achieve best fit, (2) reversibility of the procedure, and (3) absence of surgical risk. Kevin was referred to our Craniofacial Disorders Team. The team was asked to consider recommendation of a lift.

The findings of the Craniofacial Team's evaluation included identification of a bifid uvula without evidence of a submucous cleft. Videofluoroscopy was indeterminate, but suggested possible abnormal palatal movement and adenoids slightly reduced, but within normal limits for age. Speech findings were consistent with those reported previously.

Team members did not recommend a palatal lift, based on their opinion that Kevin's articulation and the prognosis associated with developmental apraxia were too poor to suggest that management of his velopharynx would make a measurable improvement in speech. Therapy, with reconsideration for a lift in three months, was recommended.

Therapy recommendations included continuation of goals to teach articulation placement and establish "acceptable" substitutions for omitted sounds. Examples included establishing bilabial and pharyngeal fricatives to substitute for oral fricatives. These recommendations were included as a secondary aspect in Phase II and will be discussed below.

Phase II: Primary Therapy Plan

Phase II of Kevin's program consisted of 45 minutes of individual therapy, four days each week. Major goals included:

(1) Increasing the frequency and accuracy of speech and sound productions that were within his physiologic capacity.

(2) Improving intelligibility by increasing vowel length and reducing glottal stopping and rate.

Implementation of the first goal consisted of eliciting combinations of nasals /m, n/ and vowels, and, producing increasingly longer sequences. Although Kevin could produce correct /m, n/ sounds, he used them only for spontaneous speech in limited, common words. *No* was the only word in which he used /n/. Therefore, therapy began with combining CV (consonant-plus-vowel) syllables and progressed to words (e.g., *none, name, man*) and phrases (e.g., *one man, no more money*). Progress was slow (see discussion) but steady, and without marked regression at any point in the program.

As Kevin's ability to sequence nasals and vowels increased, other target sounds were introduced. Sounds were chosen on the basis of his physiologic readiness for production, and included /l, j, w/. These sounds do not require high oral air pressure and Kevin's anterior tongue, jaw, and lip function were considered adequate to support production of these targets. The nasal /ŋ/ was not chosen because testing of dorsal tongue function did not indicate readiness.

The teaching of placement for /p, b, t, d/ was begun in anticipation of recommendation for the palatal lift.

The second goal was approached through a program of modelling and reinforcement conducted in therapy and at home. The therapy technique employed in all phases of remediation was based on the eight-step task continuum for therapy with apraxic adults (Rosenbek, Lemme, Aherns, Harris, and Wertz, 1973). This method was *not* chosen because of Kevin's diagnosis of developmental apraxic. It was chosen because it provides some focus on the volitional control of speech and also emphasizes a hierarchy which yields a high rate of correct-to-incorrect responses, minimizes negative practice, and gives the clinician control of the stimulus-response mode.

Phase II: Secondary Therapy Plan

As a secondary aspect of Phase II therapy, the methods suggested by the Craniofacial Disorders Team were implemented. This approach included attempting to shape sounds from nonspeech productions and establishing fricative-like sounds. Similar techniques had been attempted in Phase I. A larger percentage of time was not given to this aspect of therapy because these compensatory "speech-like" behaviors would have to be unlearned once the velopharynx was managed. Also, the active teaching of incorrect sound patterns to a child in the process of developing speech production raised serious theoretical questions. Kevin was progressing in his primary goals, which suggested time spent in therapy was used most effectively on those goals.

Status at end of Phase II

At the end of Phase II, Kevin was using /m, n/ correctly and /l/ inconsistently in spontaneous speech. Vowels were mildly distorted. Placement for bilabial (/p,b/) and tongue-tip (/t, d/) sounds was established. The use of lip smacks and tongue clicks as sound substitutions was inconsistent. Kevin more often substituted /n/ for missing speech sounds. The use of word stress and intonation was appropriate, groping for articulator placement was absent, and glottal stopping was reduced. Nasal airflow continued consistent and severe. Kevin remained unintelligible to most people. However, familiar listeners reported marked improvements in intelligibility. Kevin's great-grandmother reported she could understand portions of his speech for the first time.

INTERVENTION: PHASE III

CA: 4-0 to 5-8.

Phase III of Kevin's treatment refers to his programming with the palatal lift. Kevin returned to the Craniofacial Clinic three months after his initial visit for reconsideration of a palatal lift. Progress of Phase II therapy was reported. The evidence that articulation could be improved was decisive in the Team's recommending a lift.

The stages of fitting the prosthesis included dental restoration, palatal desensitization (Daniel, in press), fitting of the toothbands, construction of the retainer, and a single addition in the anterior-posterior dimension. The desensitization program consisted of palatal massage for approximately ten minutes, four times per day (once in therapy and three times at home). The purpose was to reduce the gag tendency. Kevin's gag was considered normal. By the time the lift was fitted, he was able to tolerate the massage approximately half way back on the velum without gagging. An additional advantage was that the program familiarized Kevin's mother with working in his mouth. The orthodontist felt the desensitization program contributed considerably to the relative ease with which the anterior-posterior portion was added. Kevin immediately wore the lift full-time, except during meals, and tolerated re-insertion of the lift without discomfort within two weeks. Within three weeks, he did not want the lift removed and was markedly reticent about talking without it.

Therapy with the Palatal Lift

The first goal of therapy with the lift in place was to establish production of oral plosives. Stimulus items contained oral consonants and vowels with no nasals. The voiced cognates /b, d/ were more stimulable and received direct therapy. Kevin produced correct oral consonants inconsistently within a week of adding the lift. Improvement was gradual, but fluctuated. Work to stabilize control of oral—as opposed to nasal—consonants continued throughout Phase III. Improvement in the production of the unvoiced cognates /p, t/ was not evident until five to six months after the lift was added.

These findings indicate that Kevin needed to be taught to use the appliance for speech. He did not demonstrate immediate control of velopharyngeal function. Rather it was a learning process.

As Kevin improved in his production of oral plosives and nasals in separate environments, more taxing stimuli were introduced and velopharyngeal control improved. First oral-nasal, non-abutting targets (e.g. *map, pan*) were introduced, and later abutting pairs (e.g. *pump*) were drilled.

Within the first month of Phase III, Kevin began to display spontaneous "vocal play." He appeared to enjoy producing a variety of speech sound types and was observed doing so in therapy and at home while playing alone. He continued to produce this "vocal play" to some extent throughout Phase III.

As sounds and approximations of speech sounds emerged in "vocal play," they were incorporated into therapy. The approximate order was /ʃ, f, k, s, v, tʃ, dʒ, g/. The rate at which Kevin gained control of each sound production varied and overlapped. The point to be emphasized is that the palatal lift allowed for an increased sound repertoire. Individual therapy targets continued to be chosen, based on Kevin's demonstration of physiologic readiness. Thus, some typically later-developing sounds received direct therapy before those usually considered as early-developing sounds.

Direct attention was given to reducing his rate of speech. A slow rate was necessary for Kevin to maintain precision and correct oral-nasal contrasts, and to reduce sound omissions and glottal stops.

Status at end of Phase III

At the end of Phase III, Kevin could produce all English speech sounds adequately, with the exception of /ŋ, r/.

Errors produced on a single word articulation test included: *inconsistent* sibilant distortion, devoicing, hypo/hypernasality, frication of stops, and developmental type errors (/f/ θ, d/ ð, w/ r, and blend simplification). In connected speech those errors were noted, as well as inconsistent sound omissions and difficulty sequencing multisyllabic words (see Figure 1).

AERODYNAMIC TESTING

Following the fitting of the lift, aerodynamic procedures were used to document that the lift size was optimal (LaVelle and Hardy, 1979). Aerodynamic findings guided the orthodontist in decisions regarding the need for change in lift size. Continued aerodynamic testing with the lift in place quantified and confirmed Kevin's perceived increase in velopharyngeal control. Test results with the lift removed indicated improved velopharyngeal function, including instances of complete closure. This could have resulted from improved velopharyngeal function secondary to wearing of the lift, delayed development of velar function, or both.

INTELLIGIBILITY

The single most important goal of Kevin's remediation program was to increase his intelligibility.

Kevin's speech prior to Phase I was rated by familiar listeners (e.g., family members) and those unfamiliar with his speech. This latter group included the examiners who treated him initially and naive listeners who rated a videotaped sample. Prior to treatment, the intelligibility ratings were similar for both types of listeners. Kevin's speech was rated between three and five percent intelligible. His use of speech was not considered functional, and he relied on gesturing to communicate. His intelligibility was essentially unchanged following Phase I of therapy.

By the end of Phase II, Kevin was still unintelligible to strangers. At that time he could produce correctly only six English consonants. Intelligibility to those close to him had increased to approximately forty to fifty percent in context. Kevin was understood more often because he was making articulatory placement, using some substitutions rather than omissions, and had reduced his speaking rate and frequency of glottal stop usage. At this point, personnel conducting his sign language program decided speech production had improved enough to warrant discontinuation of that program.

Six months after receiving the lift, Kevin had increased his intelligibility to the point of being understood in context by most listeners. He was placed in a preschool class with normal children and his speech did not hinder his progress in the classroom. By late Phase III, Kevin demonstrated correct production of all consonants except $/\eta, r/$.

Intelligibility ratings of post-therapy speech were again similar for familiar and unfamiliar listeners. His speech is considered eighty to ninety percent intelligible. His mother said he can make himself understood in all situations.

DISCUSSION

What caused this child's speech disorder? His history indicates that he had reduced strength secondary to a heart defect for his first two years of life. Descriptions of poor breath support and evidence of velopharyngeal insufficiency prior to age two suggest Kevin may not have had subglottal pressure and oral air pressure to develop normal, early speech patterns. We suspect the lack of speech production in early childhood was a major contributing factor to his speech deficit. We suggest that the motor activity of speech must be practiced in order for the neuromotor control of speech to be established in a developing child. Kevin's lack of speech without deficits in cognitive or receptive language skills is consistent with this view.

Once Kevin's heart was repaired and strength for respiratory support was present, he did not automatically begin producing all the sounds available to him (despite poor velopharyngeal function). The graph in Figure 12-2 illustrates that production of /n/ required much teaching and practice before Kevin was able to produce the sound automatically and accurately. This again suggests the necessity of practice in learning speech production.

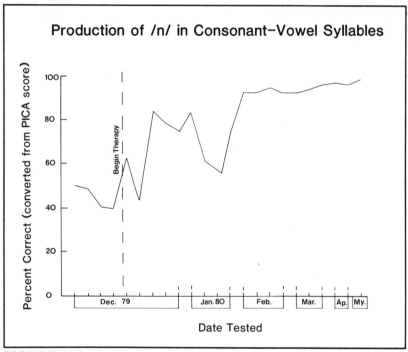

FIGURE 12-2

Measurement of progress in /n/ productions, using Base-10 procedures
Expressed as percent correct converted from PICA scores. See LaPointe (1978) for explanation of procedure.

Although Kevin did present many behaviors considered indicative of apraxia, they can be accounted for on the basis of peripheral limitations, viz., velopharyngeal incompetency and the lack of motor skill, rather than a deficit in motor programming. Kevin's limited phonological repertoire is an example.

The presence of struggle to speak, groping for correct production, and poor progress in therapy may be attributed to the clinician expecting speech beyond his motoric capacity at that time.

To determine Kevin's ability to initiate and sequence speech sounds, it was necessary to determine his peripheral abilities and test speech motor programming skills within those limits. In fact, when stimuli of only nasals and vowels were used, Kevin was able to produce sequences, did not struggle, and made progress in therapy. Consequently the diagnostic label of developmental apraxia was removed.

In addition to sorting out a complex set of presenting problems, the ongoing assessment of separate speech motor components guided therapy throughout the program. Target sounds were chosen based on what physical movements were necessary for production and the child's own capacity to produce them.

Speech and medical personnel were unable to determine the cause of the velopharyngeal incompetence, although structural abnormalities were ruled out. Had a cause been known, management of the velopharyngeal incompetence may have been initiated with less hesitation. By the beginning of Phase II, it was evident that velopharyngeal function had not changed for speech purposes and that it was having a negative effect on the use of other components. The recommendation for a lift was a pragmatic and conservative approach to management. An initial concern regarding use of the lift was the child's age. The Craniofacial Disorders Team had had children older than Kevin fail to tolerate a lift. The successful use of the lift in this case is attributed to the combined use of desensitization, parent education, and a cooperative effort between the orthodontist/prostho-dontist, speech pathologist, and family. Parent education, in addition to teaching the desensitization procedure, included an explanation of velo-pharyngeal functioning and the consequences of its malfunction, describing a lift with a model and pictures, explaining each step in the process of construction, and identifying the pros and cons of wearing a lift. It is essential that the parents and professionals working with a palatal lift candidate understand that it is not a panacea. Kevin's case shows the need for therapy in order the achieve maximum benefit from the appliance. This therapy applies to many adults as well.

The possibility of improved velopharyngeal muscle function is a consideration in choosing a lift over a surgical procedure. Careful documentation of the lift's effect is necessary to make decisions for the individual, as well as contributing information to the literature to establish prognostic information.

SUMMARY

To sum up, Kevin's story should be helpful in future speech therapy with preschool and school-aged children. His lack of progress in conventional language therapy, and with the use of nose plugs, led his clinicians to teach "compensatory articulations" and seriously consider nonverbal means of communication for him. Procedures used with adult neurogenic clients were then applied over a period of approximately 18 months and his speech became intelligible. We will never know how intelligible Kevin would have been today without this intervention. We do believe these procedures were instrumental in his talking by the time he entered school, and that other speech-handicapped children will benefit from them as well.

GLOSSARY

Tetralogy of Fallot. A combination of congenital cardiac defects consisting of pulmonary stenosis, interventricular septal defect, dextroposition of the aorta so that it overrides the interventricular system and receives venous as well as arterial blood, and right ventricular hypertrophy.

Aerodynamic Procedures. Transduction and recording of (a) intra-oral air pressure, which is the pressure recorded behind the major construction in the upper airway (in this case, the lips), and (b) volume velocity of nasal air flow.

Palatal Lift. An applicance consisting of a hard palate retainer portion with hooks that attach to the individual's teeth and a posterior extension that elevates the soft palate to the posterior pharyngeal wall. In this case, the lift was made of acrylic materials.

Palatal Desensitization. Program of palatal massage applied systematically to increase tolerance of pressure on the velum and reduce gag tendency.

Physiologic Readiness. A general term to imply that the speaker probably has adequate neurologic and musculoskeletal systems to learn the movement pattern required for the speech sound(s) of interest. Some part, or parts, of the desired movement(s) already may have been observed. If the movement(s) have never been observed by the clinician, close approximations to them should be elicited within a few therapy sessions.

REFERENCES

Daniel, B. A soft palate desensitization procedure for selected patients requiring palatal lift prosthesis. *Journal of Prosthetic Dentistry*, in press.

Jamieson, J., Matsko, T., Snyder, B., & Riegger, W. Nose plugs as a prosthetic management technique for ataxic dysarthria. Paper presented to the American Speech-Language-Hearing Association convention, Los Angeles, 1981.

LaPointe, L. Aphasia therapy: Some principles and strategies for treatment. In D. Johns (Ed.), *Clinical management of neurogenic communicative disorders.* Boston: Little, Brown & Co., 1978.

LaVelle, W., & Hardy. Palatal lift prosthesis for treatment of palatopharyngeal incompetence. *Journal of Prosthetic Dentistry*, 1979, *42*, 308-315.

Netsell, R., & Rosenbek, J. *Understanding and treating the dysarthrias.* Philadelphia: W.B. Saunders Co., in preparation.

Rosenbek, J., Lemme, M., Aherns, M., Harris, E., & Wertz, R. A treatment for apraxia of speech in adults. *Journal of Speech and Hearing Disorders*, 1973, *38*, 462-472.

ACKNOWLEDGEMENT

We wish to thank Carole Dugan for her assistance in preparation of this manuscript.

13

DAF Speech Rate Modification in Parkinson's Disease: A Report of Two Cases

Wayne R. Hanson

E. Jeffrey Metter

The speech disturbance resulting from Parkinson's disease has been described as a hypokinetic form of dysarthria (Darley, Aronson, and Brown, 1969). Hypokinetic dysarthria differs from other types of dysarthria in the extent of variability in speaking rate that is characteristic of the disorder. Dysarthric speakers generally have speaking rates that are slower than normal speakers, whereas persons with hypokinetic dysarthria may display normal, slower, or more rapid than normal rates (Canter, 1963; Darley et al. 1969). The presence of abnormally rapid rates of speech in Parkinsonian dysarthria have been documented by many writers (Netsell, Daniel, and Celesia, 1975; Mysak, 1976; Hirose, Kiritani, Ushijima, Yoshioka, and Sawashima, 1981). The data reported by Netsell et al. (1975) suggested that a possible underlying pathophysiologic mechanism affecting speech in Parkinsonism is an acceleration and weakness of specific neuromuscular control signals. When rate is particularly fast, articulatory gestures are incomplete, and some imprecision in consonant articulation usually occurs. In our experience, Parkinson's patients with extremely rapid rates present one of the most difficult challenges to successful management by the speech clinician. The primary goals of speech therapy in these cases are to control the speech rate and to increase the individual's background effort in order to achieve a more complete excursion of each articulator to its target point. With this approach, articulatory accuracy and precision are improved, and gains in speech intelligibility can occur. Unfortunately, the carry-over of improved speaking performance outside of the treatment sessions appears to be poor for many patients with Parkinson's disease (Sarno, 1968). Gaining control of accelerated speaking rate is difficult for most patients to achieve and, unfortunately, clinical strategies for rate control for these patients has received little attention in the literature. Darley, Aronson, and Brown (1975) have observed secondary gains in speaking performance resulting from the slowing of speech rate; they indicate that rate control therapy may simultaneously correct a loudness problem by concentrating greater amounts of energy in shorter speech segments. Interestingly, Netsell et al. (1975) noted that when their Parkinson's patient was asked to speak louder, acceleration behavior was reduced and his articulation became more precise. An apparent reduction in loudness has been reported as a symptom of Parkinsonian dysarthria by many writers (Canter, 1963; Boshes, 1966; Sarno, 1968; Espir and Rose, 1970). In our experience, Parkinson's patients with rapid speech rate usually present weak vocal intensity as well.

Delayed auditory feedback (DAF) has received increasing attention as a method of rate control for patient with hypokinetic dysarthria since an earlier report by Hanson and Drake (1976). Rosenbek and LaPointe (1978) have reported that DAF may have a beneficial effect on the articulation and prosody of some patients with hypokinetic dysarthria. Their clinical experience indicates that DAF appears to have its major influence on articulation time, although loudness, pitch, and prosody may also be influenced. These authors suggest that DAF may become the core of a rate modifying therapy in which the goal is to gradually wean the patient away from the DAF instrument while attempting to preserve any improvements in speech that may have been produced. In 1980, we reported data describing the effects of DAF on the speech rate, vocal intensity, and speech intelligibility of a patient with progressive supranuclear palsy (Hanson and Metter, 1980). Our patient had hypokinetic dysarthria characterized by rapid speaking rate, weak vocal intensity, and imprecise consonant articulation. This 59-year-old male was fitted with a small, wearable DAF device which he used daily for a period of three months after traditional speech therapy had produced no improvement in speech. When the device was activated (100 msec DAF), there occurred a slowing of speech rate, an increase in vocal intensity, and an improvement in speech intelligibility. Because of the similarity of this patient's clinical symptoms to those of Parkinson's disease, the authors speculated that perhaps some Parkinson's patients might experience a similar benefit from this form of intervention. Our purpose is to report the effects of DAF—produced by a small device worn daily for a period of 3 months—on the speech of two patients with Parkinson's disease and hypokinetic dysarthria. Of primary interest in this study was the influence DAF might have on the excessively rapid speaking rates exhibited by both of the subjects in this report. Further, measures of vocal intensity, fundamental frequency, and speech intelligibility are reported in order to more completely describe the influence of DAF on the speech of these dysarthic speakers.

METHOD

Subjects

Characteristics of the two patients in this report are presented in Table 13-1. At the outset of the study each patient received a neurological examination which included a rating of overall disability resulting from Parkinson's disease (Webster Rating Scale)[1]. Both patients were receiving anti-Parkinsonian medication which was not altered during the course of this study. Audiometric testing indicated normal hearing sensitivity bilaterally in each case.

Patient A., a 58-year-old man with a 3-year history of the disease, was rated as mild in overall disability. He had no detectable rigidity or tremor and his gait and posture were normal. A mild bradykinesia was present evidenced by some difficulty in handling tools and buttoning clothes. His handwriting was micrographic. Some facial immobility was apparent by a lack of facial expression, and staring. His speech intelligibility was poor as a result of hypokinetic dysarthria, characterized primarily by weak vocal intensity and excessively rapid speaking rate. Monopitch and monoloudness were also prominent in his speech. The patient had received speech therapy for a period of approximately nine months beginning one year after the onset of the Parkinson's disease. Various rate control strategies were employed during the course of speech therapy with some success during treatment sessions. However, carryover of improved speaking performance outside the clinic was not successful.

Patient B., a 56-year-old woman, first experienced the symptoms of Parkinson's disease nine years prior to the beginning of this study. The neurological examination and rating of the Parkinson's disease indicated moderate-to-severe disability. She presented marked rigidity of the neck and shoulders and some tremor in both upper extremities at rest. She was unable to swing either arm, and a moderate bradykinesia was present in both hands. Samples of her handwriting revealed severe micrographia. Her gait was shortened in stride, and there was detectable onset of simian posture with head flexed forward. She displayed moderate facial immobility and hypokinetic dysarthria characterized by rapid speech rate,

monopitch, occasionally weak vocal intensity, some imprecision in consonant articulation, and mildly impaired speech intelligibility. She had not
received speech therapy prior to this study.

TABLE 13-1
Description of two patients with Parkinson's disease

	Sex	Age	Duration of Parkinson' Disease	Neurologists' Rating of Overall Disability*	Overall Severity of Dysarthria
Patient A	Male	58	3 yrs.	Mild	Severe
Patient B	Female	56	9 yrs.	Moderate/Severe	Moderate

* Webster Rating Scale

Procedures

The DAF instrument[2] used in this study was described in our previous
report (Hanson and Metter, 1980). It's a small battery-powered device that
receives incoming audio signals from a microphone positioned near the patient's mouth. The signal delay is selected by the user (20-200 milliseconds)
and delivered to earphones located in or on the patient's ears. The device
has a loudness control, and the body of the instrument can be carried in
the pocket of a shirt or blouse.

Measurements of speaking rate, vocal intensity, fundamental frequency,
overall speech intelligibility, and phonation time for the vowel /a/ were
made from tape-recorded speech samples spoken by each subject with and
without delayed auditory feedback. Recordings were made at the beginning of treatment and at one-month intervals thereafter for a period of
three months. A total of four recording sessions was completed for each
patient. The patients wore the DAF daily, as needed, for a period of three
months. The speech samples consisted of readings of the Grandfather
Passage (Darley et al., 1975), approximately one minute of conversation
("The Job Task," from Williams, Darley, and Spriesterbach, 1978) and
maximum sustained phonation of the vowel /a/. Recordings were made
with each subject seated in a sound-treated test room (IAC Model 403A)
directly in front of a microphone (Electrovoice Model RE-15) coupled to
an Ampex tape recorder (AF 600B), located in an adjacent test room. The
mouth-to-microphone distance was 8 inches. A comfort loudness level for
DAF was determined for each patient and that level was maintained for all

recordings. The amount of delay selected for both subjects was the same, 150 milliseconds, and this setting was used for all recordings. This amount of delay was selected because, for each patient, it appeared to produce the greatest amount of slowing with the least disruption of speech flow, and both patients tolerated it well.

Rate Measurement — A measurement of overall speaking rate in words per minute (WPM) was computed for each reading of the Grandfather Passage. The number of words in each sample was divided by the number of seconds required to read the passage aloud, and that number was multiplied by 60 to give the overall speaking rate. For samples of conversation, sentence rates (WPM) were obtained using the formula described by Williams, Darley, and Spriestersbach (1978).[3] The sentence rates were then summed and divided by the total number of sentences to determine the mean sentence rate in words per minute. For the conversational speech of our patients, mean sentence rate more closely represents their actual speed of utterance exclusive of pauses and non-speaking intervals. However, mean sentence rates for conversation with normal auditory feedback were not computed for Patient A because, in many instances, individual words could not be differentiated, due to his extraordinarily rapid speaking rate and poor intelligibility.

Voice Intensity Measurement — Measures of vocal intensity were obtained by playing each speech sample into a high speed level recorder (Bruel and Kjaer Model 2305) and measuring the intensity peak in each of ten segments of equal length relative to a baseline of known sound pressure level. These values were averaged, yielding the mean peak sound pressure level (dB), which served to describe the intensity level for a particular speech sample.

Fundamental Frequency Measurement — Each recorded speech sample was played into a microprocessor-controlled fundamental frequency analyzer (Pitch Analyzer [PM 301], Voice Identification, Inc.) that automatically extracts the fundamental frequency. For each completed speech sample, the selected fundamental frequencies (128 samples per second) are stored, and the mean and standard deviation of these are computed and available as a digital display on a TV monitor. Thus, for each connected speech sample recorded in this study, a mean fundamental frequency and standard deviation was determined.

Intelligibility Measurement — Intelligibility was defined as overall understandability of speech in each connected speech sample. Median estimates of overall speech intelligibility were derived from listener ratings of each speech sample using a 7-point equal-appearing intervals scale on which 1 represented normal intelligibility and 7 represented severe deviation from normal (Darley, et al., 1969). Separate listening tapes were prepared for each subject consisting of 16 connected speech samples (8 samples of the Grandfather Passage and 8 samples of conversation), plus 6 samples repeated for reliability measurement. Three speech pathologists served as judges to rate independently the speech intelligibility of each sample. The median of the three judges' ratings was used as an index of the intelligibility for each speech sample. A total of 44 samples was rated by each judge (32 samples, plus 12 repeated for reliability). The samples for each patient were rated separately by each individual judge. When percentages of intrajudge agreement (± 1 scale value) for the two ratings of the 12 reliability samples (6 for patient A, 6 for patient B) were obtained, the lowest percentage of intrajudge agreement was 92%. The interjudge agreement (± 1 scale value) for the original 32 speech samples was 97%. A correlation of r = .96 was obtained for comparisons between the first and second ratings for each sample in the reliability group.

RESULTS

Patient A

The results of the analysis of tape-recorded speech samples of reading and conversation by patient A are presented in Tables 13-2 and 3, respectively. Statistical comparisons between the measures obtained with normal auditory feedback (NAF) and delayed auditory feedback (DAF) were made, using the t-test for correlated observations (paired). As previously mentioned, Patient A presented extremely rapid speaking rate as a primary function of his dysarthria. This feature was particularly apparent when reading aloud. The overall speaking rates for reading without delay, shown in Table 13-2, are all in excess of the rate one would expect for normal speakers.

Fairbanks (1960) has indicated a median overall speaking rate for reading by normal speakers of 170 WPM. The range for normal speaking rate for reading has been reported by Canter (1963) and Boshes (1966) as 140 to 219 WPM and 160 to 205 WPM, respectively. Patient A exceeded the range for normal speaking rate at each session with normal auditory feedback (NAF). Delayed auditory feedback (DAF) produced a marked slowing of speaking rate at each of the four sessions (t = 9.49; df = 3; p<.01). Table 13-2 shows that when 150 msec of DAF was introduced, the speaking rate for reading was slowed to a rate slightly below the range reported for normal speakers by Canter (1963). This finding was observed on the first day of treatment and at each session thereafter for a period of three months. Daily use of the DAF device during this period did not result in any noticeable carry-over of the reduction of speech rate when DAF was

TABLE 13-2

Overall speaking rate, mean peak intensity, mean fundamental frequency, and median rating of intelligibility for readings of the Grandfather Passage by Patient A

	Normal Auditory Feedback (NAF)				Delayed Auditory Feedback (DAF, 150m/sec)			
Session*	Rate** (WPM)	Intensity** (dB/SPL)	Fundamental Frequency (Hz)	Intelligibility** (1-7 pt. scale, 1 being normal)	Rate (WPM)	Intensity (dB/SPL)	Fundamental Frequency (Hz)	Intelligibility (1-7 pt. scale, 1 being normal)
1	255	65.6	103	5.00	139	72.3	150	2.00
2	233	67.7	135	6.00	122	79.7	127	3.00
3	283	65.0	115	6.00	137	77.8	115	3.00
4	226	66.7	113	6.00	139	79.3	115	2.00

* A one-month interval separates each consecutive session.
** Statistical comparison between NAF and DAF using the t-test for correlation measures (two-sided) was significant at P < .01.

not used. Overall speaking rates for reading with normal feedback remained abnormally rapid throughout the measurement interval.

As noted earlier, speaking rates for conversation with normal auditory feedback were not calculated for Patient A. Our clinical impression was that his speech in conversation with DAF was extraordinarily rapid and a marked slowing occurred with DAF. In Table 13-3, conversational speaking rates (mean sentence rates) with DAF are presented. Although information regarding mean sentence rates for normal speakers is lacking, Kelly and Steer (1949) have reported the average mean sentence rate for the extempore speech of college students as 209 WPM. The average of the mean sentence rates for Patient A, with DAF, was 166 WPM. The slowing of speech with delayed auditory feedback was observed at the beginning of treatment and at each session thereafter for a period of three months.

At the outset, Patient A exhibited very weak vocal intensity. The mean peak sound pressure levels for readings of the Grandfather Passage and for conversation were consistent with our clinical impression and are displayed in Tables 13-2 and 3. With normal auditory feedback while reading, his speech shows mean peak intensity levels that are below the lowest mean peak intensity level (72.0 dB) reported by Canter (1963) for both his Parkinson group and his normal control group. The average mean peak intensity for reading (NAF) by Patient A was 66.3 dB—the median mean peak intensity reported for normal speakers by Canter (1963) was 78.5 dB. The data show that while reading with delayed auditory feedback (150 msec) there was a significant increase in vocal intensity for each session ($t = 7.59; p < .01$). The average mean peak intensity for reading with DAF was 77.3 dB. Each of the intensity measures with DAF are within the range of intensities (72.0 - 85.9 dB) reported for normal speakers by Canter.

Table 13-3 shows that mean peak intensity for conversation also increased with the introduction of 150 msec of delayed auditory feedback ($t = 9.06; p < .01$). For conversation, the average mean peak intensity for the NAF condition was 68.9 dB and, for DAF, the average mean peak intensity was 73.1 dB. Comparison of the figures in Tables 13-2 and 3 reveals that the mean peak intensities shown are similar for both reading and conversation. No trend was noted for increased intensity over time without DAF.

The average mean fundamental frequency for reading (Table 13-2) with normal auditory feedback was 116.5 Hz and with delayed auditory feedback it was 126.8 Hz. For conversation (Table 13-3) the average of the mean fundamental frequencies was 123.5 Hz with NAF and 133.5 Hz with DAF. Although there was a tendency for fundamental frequency to increase when speaking with DAF, for reading and conversation this was not

TABLE 13-3
Mean sentence speaking rate, mean peak intensity, mean fundamental frequency, and median rating of intelligibility for conversation by Patient A

| Session | Normal Auditory Feedback (NAF) | | | | Delayed Auditory Feedback (DAF, 150m/sec) | | | |
	Rate** (WPM)	Intensity** (dB/SPL)	Fundamental Frequency (Hz)	Intelligibility** (1-7 pt. scale)	Rate (WPM)	Intensity (dB/SPL)	Fundamental Frequency (Hz)	Intelligibility 1-7 pt. scale
1	—	69.2	108	6.00	202	74.2	138	2.00
2	—	69.2	119	6.00	170	73.8	141	3.00
3	—	67.8	134	7.00	143	71.5	126	4.00
4	—	69.7	133	7.00	149	72.7	129	3.00

* Mean sentence rate with normal auditory feedback could not be measured.

** p < .01

noted consistently for each session. Fundamental frequency differences between NAF and DAF were not statistically significant (p ⟩ .05) for either reading or conversation. Patient A's average mean fundamental frequency for reading (116.5 Hz) with normal auditory feedback is below that reported for other males with Parkinson's disease and of similar age by Canter, of 129 Hz, and by Kammermeier (1969), of 130.4 Hz. The median fundamental frequency level for oral reading by normal males in the middle-age group studied by Mysak (1959) was 113.2 Hz.

Median estimates of intelligibility presented in Table 13-2 reveal, for reading with normal auditory feedback, that speech intelligibility for Patient A was grossly impaired. With delayed auditory feedback a significant improvement in speech intelligibility was noted at each of the four sessions (t = 12.99;p ⟨ .01). The average median rating for all reading samples recorded at four sessions without the benefit of DAF was 5.75. The average median rating with DAF was 2.50. Table 13-3 contains the median intelligibility ratings for conversation. The average median rating with NAF was 6.50, and, with DAF the average median rating was 3.00. The differences in intelligibility ratings between normal and delayed auditory feedback were significant (t = 12.12;p ⟨ .01).

TABLE 13-4
Phonation times for the vowel /a/

	Patient A		Patient B	
Session	*NAF* * *(seconds)*	*DAF* *(150/msec)* *(seconds)*	*NAF* *(seconds)*	*DAF* *(150/msec)* *(seconds)*
1	20.9	24.9	5.0	7.2
2	17.3	22.8	6.2	6.0
3	26.0	28.9	5.2	5.2
4	35.4	34.2	7.2	7.4

*Normal auditory feedback

Phonation times for the vowel /a/ are reported for Patient A in Table 13-4. Darley et al. (1975) have indicated that the ability to sustain vowel phonation is a measure that may serve as a vehicle for assessing respiratory support for speech. A reduced ability to sustain vowel phonation by Parkinson's patients has been reported by Canter (1963). His group of Parkinson patients (mean age 56 years, 10 months) had a median phonation time for the vowel /a/ of 9.5 seconds. His normal control group had a median phonation time of 20.6 seconds. Boshes (1966) reported mean phonation times of 11.7 seconds for Parkinson patients and 25.1 seconds for matched normal subjects. Somewhat contradictory findings were reported by Kreul (1972), who found that a group of 23 Parkinsonian patients (mean age 56 years) was able to prolong the vowel /a/ an average of 20.5 seconds. Patient A had a mean phonation time for /a/ of 24.9 seconds with normal auditory feedback and a mean of 27.7 seconds with DAF. Thus, Patient A appears to be well within the range of normal speakers in ability to sustain vowel phonation. There appears to be no consistent effect of DAF on phonation time for the vowel /a/ by Patient A.

Patient B

Patient B had complained of a gradual increase in speaking rate following the onset of Parkinson's disease. The clinical impression of excessively rapid speech was confirmed by the results of this study. Her speaking rates for reading aloud are shown in Table 13-5. The mean speaking rate for reading with normal auditory feedback was 183.25 words per minute. This rate exceeds the median speaking rates for normal speakers reported by Fairbanks (1960) of 170 WPM and Canter (1963), 177.6 WPM. Although the subjects in Canter's study were male, and our Patient B female, Johnson (1961) has reported no significant differences in rate of oral reading and speaking between male and female subjects. When the DAF instrument was used and Patient B read aloud, her overall speaking rates were slowed significantly (t = 4.67; p < .05). The mean overall speaking rate for reading aloud with DAF was 137.25 WPM. In Table 13-5, it can be seen that a slowing of speaking rate for conversation occurred when DAF was used (t = 3.29; p < .05). Her mean speaking rate for conversation with normal auditory feedback was 238.8 WPM, and the rate with DAF was 166.8 WPM. Without DAF, speaking rates for reading and conversation remained excessively rapid during the entire period of this study.

The mean peak intensities for reading aloud and conversation by Patient B are presented in Table 13-5 and 13-6, respectively. In all instances except session 3 (conversation), mean peak intensity with DAF exceeds the intensity levels for samples spoken with normal auditory feedback. With delayed auditory feedback, there was an increase in mean peak intensity for both reading and conversation. However, only for reading was the increase statistically significant (t = 4.75, p < .05). Interestingly, although the authors clinically perceived that Patient B presented with weak vocal intensity, the data show that she was within the range of intensity that would be expected for normal speakers (72.0 dB-89.5 dB; Canter, 1963) for reading aloud. The average mean peak intensity for reading with normal auditory feedback was 75.5 dB and the average intensity for conversation was 76.5 dB.

TABLE 13-5
Overall speaking rate, mean peak intensity, mean fundamental frequency and median rating of intelligibility for reading aloud by Patient B

	Normal Auditory Feedback (NAF)				Delayed Auditory Feedback (DAF, 150m/sec)			
Session	Rate* (WPM)	Intensity* (dB/SPL)	Fundamental** Frequency (Hz)	Intelligibility (1-7 pt. scale)	Rate (WPM)	Intensity (dB/SPL)	Fundamental Frequency (Hz)	Intelligibility (1-7 pt. scale)
1	184	77.3	206	2.00	122	79.1	215	2.00
2	184	73.6	196	3.00	120	77.1	210	2.00
3	176	76.0	184	2.00	149	77.3	197	1.00
4	189	75.2	192	2.00	158	77.6	206	1.00

*p < .05
**p < .01

TABLE 13-6
Mean sentence speaking rate, mean peak intensity, mean fundamental frequency and median rating of intelligibility for conversation by Patient B

	Normal Auditory Feedback (NAF)				Delayed Auditory Feedback (DAF, 150m/sec)			
Session	Rate* (WPM)	Intensity (dB/SPL)	Fundamental Frequency (Hz)	Intelligibility* (1-7 pt. scale)	Rate (WPM)	Intensity (dB/SPL)	Fundamental Frequency (Hz)	Intelligibility 1-7 pt. scale
1	242	77.6	207	3.00	161	81.2	209	2.00
2	282	72.7	191	4.00	152	78.2	206	3.00
3	231	79.3	184	3.00	188	79.0	188	2.00
4	200	76.6	196	4.00	166	80.8	206	2.00

*p < .05

The data reported in Table 13-5 reveal that, for reading aloud, mean fundamental frequency increased significantly (t = 10.50;p < .01) with delayed auditory feedback. The average mean fundamental frequency for reading was 194.5 Hz when Patient B spoke with normal auditory feedback. The mean speaking fundamental frequency reported recently for normal nonsmoking females in the 50-59 age group was 199.3 Hz (Stoicheff, 1981). In Table 13-5, it can be seen that although slight increases occurred in mean fundamental frequency for conversation with DAF, these increases were not statistically significant. The average mean fundamental frequency for conversation with normal feedback was identical to that obtained for reading aloud (194.5 Hz).

The median estimates of intelligibility scores for reading are shown in Table 13-5. It can be seen that these scores increased slightly (except in session 1) with DAF. Intelligibility scores for conversation are reported in Table 13-6. The increases in intelligibility scores for conversation with DAF were greater than those for reading, and were statistically significant (t = 4.99;p < .05). Comparison of the median ratings of intelligibility in Tables 13-5 and 13-6 indicates that, with normal auditory feedback, Patient B showed greater impairment in conversation than in oral reading.

Referring back to Table 13-4, the ability of Patient B to sustain vowel phonation appeared to be severly impaired. The phonation time for the vowel /a/ that would be expected for a normal female speaker of her age (58 years) is approximately 15 seconds. Kreul (1972) has reported a mean duration for prolonged vowel phonation (/a/) by elderly females (mean age 70.8 years) of 14.6 seconds. A younger group (mean age 21 years) was able to prolong the vowel /a/ for a mean of 18.2 seconds. Interestingly, Kreul also reported a mean phonation time for /a/ for a group of Parkinson patients (mean age 55.8 years) as being 20.5 seconds. Patient B had a mean phonation time for /a/ with normal auditory feedback of 5.9 seconds. The mean phonation time for /a/ with DAF was 6.45 seconds. DAF did not appear to influence the time of maximum sustained vowel phonation for Patient B.

DISCUSSION

Normally, variations in speaking rate are accomplished by altering the number and extent of pauses in connected discourse (Minifie, 1973). With delayed auditory feedback most speakers experience a slowing of speaking rate resulting from increases in both articulation time and pause time (Burke, 1975). The Parkinson patients in this report showed a marked reduction in speech rate under DAF. To further demonstrate the influence of DAF on these speakers, tracings of a phrase from the Grandfather Passage, spoken by each patient, are displayed in Figures 13-1 and 2. The phrase "A long flowing beard clings to his chin" was taken from recordings made with and without DAF at one session. Outputs (fundamental frequency and relative amplitude) from the Pitch Analyzer (PM 301) were displayed simultaneously on two separate channels of a Mingograph (Model 805), operated at a paper speed of 50 mm per second. From these tracings total duration of each phrase, as well as articulation time and pause time within the phrase, was determined. Examination of the tracings reveals the extent of the increases in articulation time and pause time with DAF. Figure 13-1 shows

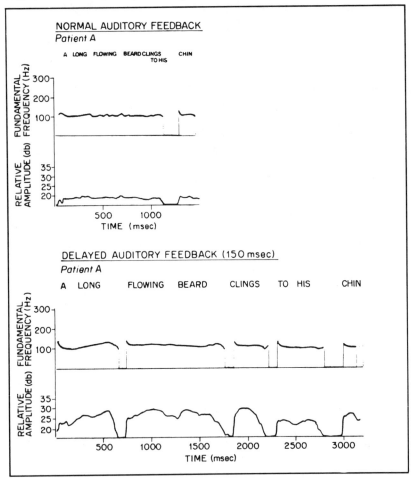

FIGURE 13-1

Fundamental frequency, relative amplitude, and duration for the phrase "A long flowing beard clings to his chin" produced with normal auditory feedback and with delayed auditory feedback by Patient A

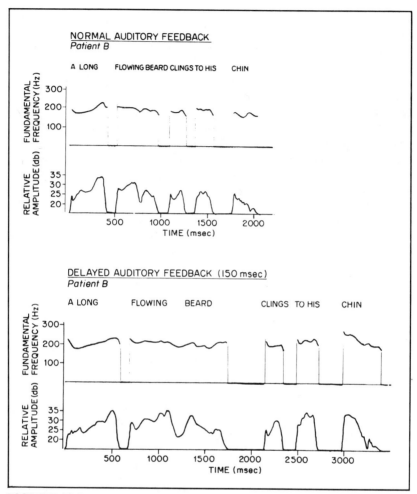

FIGURE 13-2
**Fundamental frequency, relative amplitude, and duration for the phrase
"A long flowing beard clings to his chin" produced with normal auditory
feedback and with delayed auditory feedback by Patient B**

that when Patient A spoke with normal auditory feedback, the phrase appears compressed and without distinct segmentation except for a pause before the final word in the phrase. This pattern of continuous voicing and monotone fundamental frequency appears to resemble the prosodic disturbance Kent (1979) has labeled "blurring." With DAF, there is a distinct differentiation of the segments and the between-segment pauses. For Patient B (Figure 13-2), the articulated segments and pauses are apparent for both normal and delayed auditory feedback. Of interest here is the approximately proportional increase in articulation time and pause time that occurred under DAF. With delayed feedback, total articulation time for the phrase spoken by Patient B increased from 1,480 msec to 2,480 msec and total pause time increased from 530 to 900 msec. Increases in relative amplitude and fundamental frequency with DAF are also apparent in the figures. Analysis of the suprasegmentals of time, frequency, and intensity, as displayed in these figures, suggests that alterations in the prosodic features of speech occurring with DAF may be identified using this method.

The findings for both patients suggest that when they spoke with delayed auditory feedback, their respective levels of physiological effort increased. The effects of increased physiological effort on speech are multiple. Increases in intensity and fundamental frequency may occur with increased effort. The force with which two articulators make contact for consonant production may be greater with increases in speaking effort. It has been suggested that the increase in contact force that accompanies the increase in effort is very likely the result of greater neural signal strength to the musculature (Netsell, 1973). Also, Netsell et al. (1975) observed increases in the amplitude and duration of muscle action potentials of orbicularis oris, and a reduction in acceleration behavior, when they requested their patient with Parkinson's disease to speak more loudly. These authors theorized that the increase in physiological effort associated with the increased loudness may somehow override or suppress a neural feedback circuit that is involved in the acceleration behavior. The overall rapid speech rate, short rushes of speech, or acceleration behavior occur in a neuromuscular mode over which Parkinson's patients have limited control. As speculation, it may be that the insertion of a time lag (DAF) into the neural feedback regulating mechanism not only serves to alert the nervous system, but also allows time for more efficient monitoring of feedback, and results in an increase in the neural signal strength required for increased speaking effort. Mysak (1976) has postulated that the slowing of speech resulting from DAF may allow a deficient auditory sensor system time to perform its control function more efficiently. In addition, he indicated that DAF may also cause an individual to reject the sound of his speech and to concentrate on tactile-kinesthetic feedback in altering speech output. Although our patients appeared to increase their levels of effort when speaking under DAF, increased effort did not seem to generalize to situations when they spoke without the benefit of delay.

One measure of the adequacy of the physiological support for speech is the maximum time of sustained vowel phonation. Canter (1965) found that the ability to sustain vowel phonation was correlated with the overall speech adequacy of the Parkinson's patients in his study. For the two patients in the present report phonation time for the vowel /a/ was not a good predictor of speech adequacy, nor was the overall degree of disability associated with Parkinson's disease. Patient A, with the least overall disability and normal phonation time ($\bar{x} = 24.9$ seconds) had severe speech impairment. Patient B, with moderate-to-severe overall disability and reduced phonation time ($\bar{x} = 5.9$ seconds) was much less impaired in speaking. Common to both patients, however, was a notable lack of control of speaking rate.

It has been reported that reduced pitch variability is characteristic of the patient with Parkinson's disease, and that this reduction may be partly responsible for the monotonicity of Parkinsonian speech (Canter, 1963). Because monopitch was a characteristic of the hypokinetic dysarthria presented by both patients in this study, contrasting the standard deviations for the mean fundamental frequencies obtained for speech samples spoken with and without DAF was of interest. The mean fundamental frequencies and their standard deviations are reported in Table 13-7. The size of the standard deviations for Patient B did not differ greatly between normal and delayed auditory feedback conditions, while for Patient A there was a marked difference. Increases in the size of the standard deviations were noted at each session when Patient A spoke under DAF. No further analysis of these data was undertaken.

How delayed auditory feedback can best be utilized in the clinical management of hypokinetic dysarthria must be determined by individual speech clinicians following careful assessment of the needs of a particular patient. For some patients with Parkinson's disease, particularly those with poor speech intelligibility resulting from abnormally rapid speech rate and weak vocal intensity, treatment options may be very limited. If DAF helps the patient to speak more effectively, then a trial period using a portable DAF device may be warranted. If attempts to gradually wean the patient away from the DAF instrument while maintaining improved speech are successful, then an optimal outcome has been achieved. However, the possibility that DAF may serve as a compensatory speech aid, with or without other forms of therapy, should receive consideration. The most appropriate management of speech disorders associated with progressive neurological disease requires periodic reassessment of the patient's needs. Intervention strategies may change as the needs of the patient change. Patient A, for example, after traditional speech therapy met with no success, was aided with DAF in improving speech intelligibility. Although he was permitted to continue using the wearable DAF instrument beyond the time of this study, he returned it within a few weeks indicating that he had dropped it and that it was inoperative. He was not seen again for many months and when he reappeared, the effects of the Parkinson's disease were more apparent, including a further deterioration of speech. Currently he uses a combination of DAF (a desk top model for use at home) and a hand held paper print-out device as aids to communication. Patient B continues to use the wearable DAF unit

TABLE 13-7
Mean fundamental frequency and standard deviation for reading and conversation

	Mean Fundamental Frequency (Hz) and Standard Deviation							
	Patient A				Patient B			
	NAF		DAF (150/msec)		NAF		DAF (150/msec)	
	$\overline{X}$	SD	$\overline{X}$	SD	$\overline{X}$	SD	$\overline{X}$	SD
Reading								
Session								
1	103	14	150	64	206	20	215	22
2	135	16	127	42	196	30	210	24
3	115	8	115	28	184	22	197	28
4	113	12	115	22	192	18	206	20
Conversation								
Session								
1	108	12	138	44	207	18	209	20
2	119	10	141	52	191	14	206	22
3	134	12	126	16	184	16	188	18
4	133	16	129	26	196	18	206	30

with satisfaction. She reports that the slower speaking rate with DAF is preferable to the excessively rapid rate she experiences when DAF is not used. Her husband concurs with this assessment. The relatively small improvement in overall speech intelligibility in conversation noted by the judges for Patient B is perceived as an important gain by the patient and her spouse.

NOTES

[1] David D. Webster, *Webster Rating Scale, Parkinson's Disease Patient Evaluation,* Endo Laboratories, Inc. Garden City, N.Y., 1979.

[2] Personal Speech Delay (PSD), Behavioral Controls Division of ALPS, Inc., Milwaukee, Wisconsin.

[3] Sentence Rate (WPM) = seconds $\div \dfrac{\text{sentence length in seconds}}{\text{number of words in sentence}}$

REFERENCES

Boshes,B. Voice change in Parkinsonism. *Journal of Neurosurgery,* 1966, 286-288. (Supplement 24)

Burke,. Susceptibility to delayed auditory feedback and dependence on auditory or oral sensory feedback. *Journal of Communicative Disorders,* 1975, *8*, 75-96.

Canter,G. Speech characteristics of patients with Parkinson's disease: 1. Intensity, pitch, and duration. *Journal of Speech and Hearing Disorders,* 1963, *28*, 221-229.

Canter, G. Speech characteristics of patients with Parkinson's disease: III. Articulation diadochokinesis, and overall speech adequacy. *Journal of Speech and Hearing Disorders,* 1965, *30*, 217-224.

Darley,F., Aronson,A., & Brown,J. Differential diagnostic patterns of dysarthria. *Journal of Speech and Hearing Research*, 1969, *12*, 246-269.

Darley,F., Aronson,A., & Brown,J. *Motor speech disorders.* Philadelphia: W.B. Saunders Co., 1975.

Espir,M., & Rose,F. *The basic neurology of speech.* Philadelphia: F.A. David Co., 1970.

Fairbanks,G., *Voice and articulation drillbook,* (2nd ed.). New York: Harper, 1960.

Hanson,W., & Drake,P. The use of delayed auditory feedback in the treatment of Parkinsonian dysarthria. Presentation to the American Speech-Language-Hearing Association Convention, Houston, 1976.

Hanson,W., & Metter,E. DAF as instrumental treatment for dysarthria in progressive supranuclear palsy: A case report. *Journal of Speech and Hearing Disorders,* 1980, *45,*268-276.

Hirose,H., Kiritani,S., Ushijima,T., Yoshioka,H., & Sawashima,M. Patterns of dysarthric movements in patients with Parkinsonism. *Folia Phoniatrica,* 1981, *33,* 204-215.

Johnson,W. Measurement of oral reading and speaking rate and disfluency of adult male and female stutterers and nonstutterers. *Journal of Speech and Hearing Disorders Monograph,* 1961, 1-20, (7).

Krammermeier, M. *A comparison of phonatory phenomena among groups of neurologically impaired speakers.* Doctoral dissertation, University of Minnesota, 1969.

Kelly,J., & Steer,M. Revised concept of rate. *Journal of Speech and Hearing Disorders,* 1949, *14,* 222-226.

Kent,R. Prosodic disturbance and neurologic lesion. Paper presented to the American Speech-Language-Hearing Association convention, Atlanta, 1979.

Kreul,E. Neuromuscular control examination (NMC) for Parkinsonism: Vowel prolongations and diadochokinetic and reading rates. *Journal of Speech and Hearing Research,* 1972, *15,* 72-83.

Minifie, F. Speech acoustics. In F. Minifie, T. Hixon, & F. Williams, (Eds.), *Normal aspects of speech hearing and language.* Englewood Cliffs, NJ: Prentice-Hall, 1973.

Mysak,E. Pitch and duration characteristics of older males. *Journal of Speech and Hearing Research,* 1959, *2,* 46-54.

Mysak,E. *Pathologies of speech systems.* Baltimore: Williams & Wilkins, 1976.

Netsell,R. Speech physiology. In F. Minifie, T. Hixon, & F. Williams, (Eds.), *Normal aspects of speech, hearing, and language.* Englewood Cliffs, NJ: Prentice-Hall, 1973.

Netsell,R., Daniel,B., Celesia,G. Acceleration and weakness in Parkinsonian dysarthria. *Journal of Speech and Hearing Disorders,* 1975, *40,* 170-178.

Rosenbek,J., & LaPointe,L. Dysarthria: Description, diagnosis and treatment. In D. John (Ed.), *Clinical management of neurogenic communication disorders.* Boston: Little, Brown & Co., 1978.

Sarno,M. Speech impairment in Parkinson's disease. *Archives of Physical Medicine Rehabilitation,* 1968, *49,* 269-275.

Stoicheff,M. Speaking fundamental frequency charactistics of nonsmoking female adults. *Journal of Speech and Hearing Research,* 1981, *24,* 437-440.

Williams,D., Darley,F., & Spriesterbach,D. Appraisal of rate and fluency. In F. Darley & D. Spriesterbach (Eds.), *Diagnostic methods in speech pathology* (2nd ed.), New York: Harper & Row, 1978.

14

Immediate Visual Feedback in the Treatment of Ataxic Dysarthria: A Case Study

William R. Berry

Edward L. Goshorn

Background Information

In the past, a prevalent notion among speech pathologists was that little could be done to improve the communication of an adult who suffers from chronic dysarthria. While the basis for such a generalization remains somewhat undefined, a body of literature is now being developed to alter the strategies in rehabilitation of dysarthria. Reports by clinician-researchers who have carefully documented their treatment techniques and results (Daniel and Guitar, 1978; Garber, Burzynski, Vale, and Nelson, 1979; Hand, Burns, and Ireland, 1979; Netsell and Cleeland, 1973; Netsell and Daniel, 1979) now suggest that even patients who suffer from severe chronic dysarthria can expect more positive results from treatment.

We have observed that speech therapy with dysarthric adults generally relies upon the clinician's judgment of patient responses. A more favorable treatment plan would allow the patient to monitor and change speech behaviors as efficiently as possible. A biofeedback paradigm in which the patient receives instantaneous and continuous information about his neuromotor behavior may be the most desirable for shaping behavior toward a desired goal. A number of biofeedback treatment techniques for dysarthria patients have been described (Hands, Burns, and Ireland, 1979; Daniel and Guitar, 1978, Netsell and Cleeland, 1973). These rely on clinician-patient interaction for the most part.

Another desirable technique that minimizes the patient's dependency on the therapist utilizes immediate visual feedback of speech events so that the subject can visualize and judge the adequacy of a response by predetermined criteria. Mirrors or feathers have been used to allow the dysarthric with a weak velum to see the inappropriate air flow through the nose. As Provost (1947) described, clinicians have used a VU meter on their tape recorders to allow a patient to get immediate feedback about speech intensity. Garber et al. (1979) described the use of a device to provide a patient with simultaneous visual information about vocal intensity and nasalization.

In recent years, electronic visual storage units have been developed that provide the speech clinician with an array of treatment instrumentation. In this study, a single subject design is used to illustrate the use of immediate oscillographic feedback of intensity in the treatment of a stroke victim with severe dysarthria.

METHODS

Subject

The patient, S., was a 60-year-old male who had severe ataxia from several cerebrovascular episodes six months prior to a speech evaluation. His speech was characterized by irregular articulatory imprecision, rapid/variable rate, harsh/breathy phonation, excessive loudness, and reduced intelligibility. We concluded that he had severe ataxic dysarthria (Darley, Aronson, and Brown, 1969). Prior to the referral, he received speech therapy for approximately two months where he had been hospitalized following his strokes. Reports from the patient, his wife, and the therapist indicated that treatment had been unsuccessful with a goal of improved articulatory abilities. From the case history, the severity of S.'s dysarthria, and the time post onset, the prognosis for significant improvement in intelligibility seemed poor. However, the patient indicated that he definitely wanted to improve his speech because of the embarrassment he was suffering. A clinical contract was established with the patient for approximately six weeks of treatment to be followed by a re-evaluation of intelligibility at the end of that time.

Clinical Hypothesis

From our evaluation, we had observed that S. had a tendency to "over-drive" his poorly coordinated speech system, habitually speaking too rapidly and loudly. We hypothesized that if S. could learn to slow his rate, his intelligibility would improve. Toward this goal, immediate feedback of the intensity of his speech was the treatment selected.

Recording Procedures

A randomized list of forty sentences was recorded before initiating therapy, using a high fidelity recording system (Tandberg-Series 15) in an audiometric sound suite with controls for a microphone/mouth distance, microphone/room placement, and record level. The forty sentences were random selections from the SPIN lists, constructed by experimental design to test intelligibility (Kalikow, Stevens, and Elliott, 1977). The list recorded was made up of 20 high and 20 low probability items. The list was also re-randomized and re-recorded at two subsequent intervals: (1) after 5 weeks of treatment, and, then, (2) after two weeks of no treatment(i.e., a vacation for which treatment was interrupted). All controls to standardize/control acoustic variables were exercised for each recording. On each occasion, the subject was instructed to "read the sentences as clearly as possible." S. exhibited no particular difficulty reading the sentences, but sentences were re-recorded when reading errors were made.

Treatment Procedures

Following pretherapy recording of the sentences, treatment was begun on a twice-per-week basis (forty-five minute sessions). S. was positioned within view of a storage oscilloscope (F.J. Electronics; Curve Display) pre-set to display a five-second sweep tracing. He was instructed to read or repeat sentences selected from the SPIN lists. The randomized sentences used in therapy comprised one-half, or twenty, of those used for the listening study (ten each having low and high probability). S.'s production of each sentence was channeled through an acoustic system to provide him with immediate visual information about his intensity. He spoke into a microphone held at a constant distance from his mouth. Sentences were amplified and filtered by an F.J. Electronics Intensity Meter (Model IM 360) to measure a log function of the intensity above 2 K HZ. The multicolor storage oscilloscope was used to provide S. with a method for monitoring his rate and loudness.

Before the patient spoke each sentence, the clinician recorded a model which was stored on the oscilloscope in one of the four colors available for tracing. A second color line was preset at a standard distance above the first to identify an upper limit of intensity. The patient's goal, therefore, was to keep his loudness level below the upper line and go slowly enough to "fill up" more than half of the screen on the intensity tracing. S.'s production of the sentence was displayed on the scope by a third color scan line with the loudness limit in a fourth color. S. was asked to judge his rate and loudness relative to the model. The lines limiting his intensity were simply used to maintain a constant loudness during therapy. He had a tendency to speak a bit too loudly, probably due to a moderate hearing loss. Our main interest, however, was to make S. conscious of his rate. During therapy, vertical lines were drawn at the mid-point of the time line on a plastic sheet covering the scope. S. was instructed that his sentence should go beyond this vertical line and fill up as much of the screen as possible. With each sentence, as the patient met the duration criteria, a good production was stored on the scope, and he produced that sentence several times in other colors, allowing him to visually compare his output with this own model, a technique to promote consistency of production.

Listening Procedures

The three recordings of the randomized high and low predictability sentences were presented in a counterbalanced order to twelve listeners who had no previous contact with the SPIN lists. The sentences were presented at 40 dB SL (relative to each listener's normal SRT) with white noise added at a + 10 signal-to-noise ratio. The listeners were instructed to "fill in the word that is most likely to occur at the end of the sentence" (after Kalikow, et al., 1977), and to write the word that was perceived. The listener's responses were compared to "key words" that S. intended to produce. An intelligibility score was derived by assigning one error for each omission, substitution, or addition of phonemes, and by deriving a percentage of correctly perceived phonemes of the total possible.

Rate Measurements

The standard recordings of the SPIN sentences were played through the same filter system used for feedback during therapy. To obtain a number of duration measurements from the tapes, however, an ultraviolet printout device (F.J. Electronics; Model R1200 UV Recorder) was utilized. Measures of overall sentence duration, key word duration, and total pause time for each sentence from these intensity X time tracings were obtained. As with the intelligibility data, these duration measurements were compared for the two time intervals under question—that is, for the five weeks of therapy (TIME A) and a two-week interval following treatment when the patient received no therapy (TIME B).

RESULTS

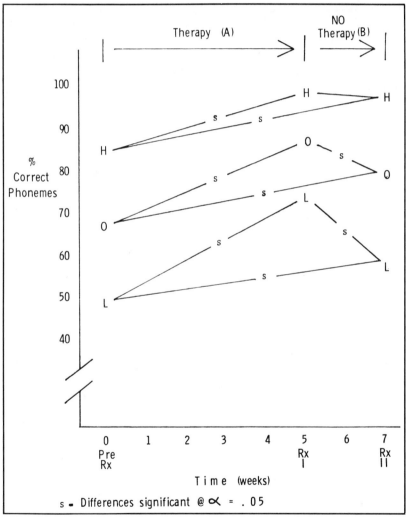

FIGURE 14-1
Summary of intelligibility over time

Figure 14-1 summarizes the mean intelligibility scores from the twelve listeners, showing the changes in intelligibility over Times A and B. Besides the overall intelligibility scores (O), the scores on the low (L) and high (H) predictability sentences are shown. These intelligibility data were subjected to statistical manipulation to measure the differences between the average score over time. (See Appendix A, Tables 1-3 for t-test results). Significant differences in average intelligibility scores were measured by a series of t-tests for all variables (i.e., H, O, L) across both time intervals, except for the high probability sentences where no difference was measured for time period B. Significant increases in H, O, and L were measured for Time A, and that except for H (Time B), there were significant decreases exhibited for the no-therapy period (B). The latter, however, did not return to previous levels as measured by the significant differences across the entire 7-week period.

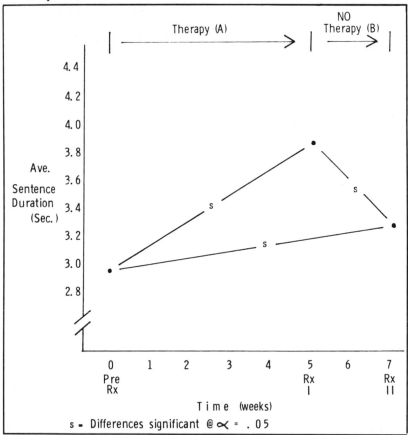

FIGURE 14-2
Average total sentence duration in seconds

The second part of our clinical hypothesis dealt with the patient's rate of speech. Figure 14-2 shows the measurements of average overall sentence duration. An increase in this measurement for Time A and a decrease over the no-therapy differences were obtained between all time intervals. (See Appendix A, Table 14-4 for t-test results.)

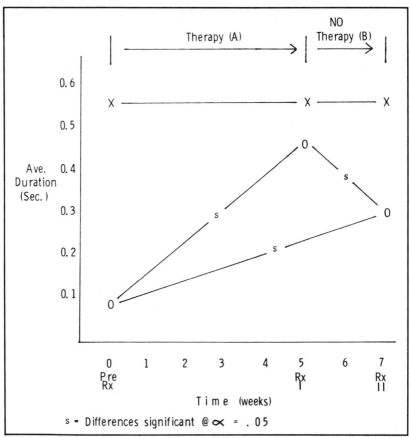

FIGURE 14-3

Average duration (sec.) of key words (X) and total pause time (O)

A number of sub-variables of rate were then measured, including the duration of the key SPIN words and average total pause time (overall and for both types of sentences). Figure 14-3 illustrates the key word duration and overall pause time as a function of the treatment periods. Here it can be seen that the significant differences in overall sentence duration (Figure 14-2) were mirrored by differences in total pause time. The average key word duraton, however, demonstrated no essential differences over time. (See Appendix A, Tables 14-5 and 14-6 for t-test results.)

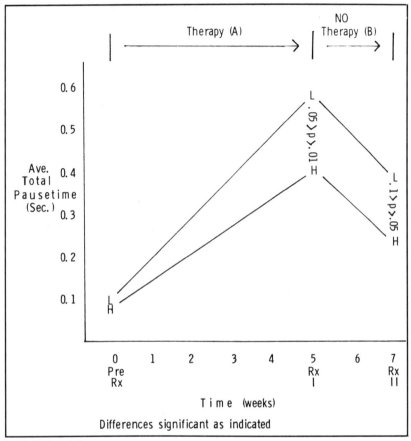

FIGURE 14-4
Average pausetime for hi/lo probability SPIN sentences in seconds

No significant differences in total pause time for the two types of SPIN sentences (lo/hi) was measured at the outset of therapy (Figure 14-4). After Time A, however, the patient produced significantly longer pauses on low probability sentences. Though the difference was less significant, a similar pattern was noted after Time B. (See Appendix A, Table 14-7 for t-test results.)

DISCUSSION

In reflecting upon these results, we feel that our investigation supports the efficacy of our treatment utilizing immediate visual feedback. For the primary five-week therapy period, our data indicate that S. did, in fact, slow his rate of speech and improve his intelligibility on the criterion task. The improvement was so apparent that one listener thought that more than one person was speaking the sentences. The patient's wife and other family members made a number of unsolicited positive remarks about his improvement which supported the clinical validity of our statistical findings.

After the first treatment period, the patient went on a two-week vacation which permitted a test of the effects of time with no therapy. Three days prior to the second post-therapy recording, however, S. apparently sustained an ischemic fainting episode. Though the wife and family did not report any speech deterioration, our data indicate that intelligibility decreased as rate of speech increased. We cannot say whether this was due to the effects of time, ischemia, or both. The patient did not resume treatment following the second post-therapy recording for personal reasons.

The findings and their apparent support of our therapy approach led to additional questions about the rate strategies spontaneously and arbitrarily developed by the subject in an effort to improve intelligibility. No specific rate strategies were taught, the subject was simply told to "go slower." He was given an immediate visual confirmation of his success or failure. Evidently S. utilized one or several components of the task to alter his speech rate.

Of additional interest was the effect of pause lengthening in S.'s speech. While producing the key words with the same average duration, S. learned to systematically prolong pauses. The speech produced with the longer pauses was found to be higher in intelligibility. In five weeks of treatment, the patient was consistent in his use of longer pauses between and/or within words, even to the point of using longer pauses in sentences which had fewer semantic cues. The latter is fascinating since S. had no conscious knowledge that low versus high probability sentences were being used in therapy. Perhaps this strategy allowed his discoordinate articulatory system more time to accurately prepare for the upcoming articulatory movements. It is also logical that the pauses allowed the listeners more time to process the information in the post-treatment sentences.

The efficacy data for treatment described and the information related to the patient's speech strategies require additional clinical and/or experimental confirmation. However, in the face of a poor prognosis, the severely dysarthric subject of this study learned to use pauses in ten sessions of exposure to immediate oscilloscopic feedback. These data are encouraging.

REFERENCES

Daniel,R., & Guitar,B. EMG feedback and recovery of facial and speech gestures following neural anastomosis. *Journal of Speech and Hearing Disorders,* 1978, *43*, 9-20.

Darley,F., Aronson,A., & Brown,J. Differential diagnostic patterns of dysarthria. *Journal of Speech and Hearing Research,* 1969, *12*, 246-269.

Garber,S., Burzynski,C., Vale,C., & Nelson,R. The use of visual feedback to control vocal intensity and nasalization. *Journal of Communicative Disorders,* 1979, 12, 399-410.

Hand,C., Burns,M. & Ireland,E. Treatment of hypertonicity in muscles of lip retraction. *Biofeedback & Self Regulation,* 1979, *4*, 171-181.

Kalikow,D., Steven,K., & Elliott,L. Development of a test of speech intelligibility in noise using sentence materials with controlled predictability. *Journal of the Acoustical Society of America,* 1977, *61*, 1337-1351.

Netsell,R., & Cleeland,C. Modification of lip hypotonia in dysarthria using EMG feedback. *Journal of Speech and Hearing Disorders,* 1973, *38*, 131-140.

Netsell,R., & Daniel,B. Dysarthria in adults: Physiologic approach to rehabilitation. *Archives of Physical Medicine and Rehabilitation,* 1979, *60* 502-508.

Provost,W. Visual aids to speech improvement. *Journal of Speech and Hearing Disorders,* 1947, *12*, 387-391.

ACKNOWLEDGEMENT

This paper was presented in a more abbreviated format at the 1979 American Speech-Language and Hearing Association Convention in Atlanta, Georgia. The authors wish to acknowledge the support of the Research and Medical Media Services at the Memphis VA Medical Center.

APPENDIX A

TABLE 14-1
Overall intelligibility differences (percentage scores)

Source	Mean	SD	t
Pre-Rx	67.85	10.04	-7.88*
Rx 1	88.20	4.34	
Rx 1	88.20	4.34	5.19*
Rx 11	78.47	6.87	
Pre-Rx	67.85	10.04	-3.82*
Rx 11	78.47	6.87	

*p<.05. df = 11 (2-tailed)

TABLE 14-2
Intelligibility differences (percentage scores) for high probability sentences

Source	Mean	SD	t
Pre-Rx	85.36	10.32	-4.87*
Rx 1	99.35	1.04	
Rx 1	99.35	1.04	1.86
Rx 11	97.43	3.50	
Pre-Rx	85.36	10.32	-4.23*
Rx 11	97.43	3.50	

*p<.05, df = 11 (2-tailed)

TABLE 14-3
Intelligibility differences (percentage scores) for low probability sentences

Source	Mean	SD	t
Pre-Rx	48.07	12.17	-9.08*
Rx 1	75.72	9.52	
Rx 1	75.72	9.52	5.60*
Rx 11	57.01	11.86	
Pre-Rx	48.07	12.17	-2.44*
Rx 11	57.01	11.86	

*p⟨.05, df = 11 (2-tailed)

TABLE 14-4
Differences in mean sentence duration (SEC.)

Source	Mean	SD	t
Pre-Rx	2.98	0.42	-12.99*
Rx 1	3.90	0.46	
Rx 1	3.90	0.46	7.47*
Rx 11	3.33	0.35	
Pre-Rx	2.98	0.42	- 5.67*
Rx 11	3.33	0.35	

*p⟨.05, df = 39 (2-tailed)

TABLE 14-5
Differences in mean key word duration (SEC.)

Source	Mean	SD	t
Pre-Rx	0.587	0.163	1.345
Rx 1	0.569	0.145	
Rx 1	0.569	0.145	0.197
Rx 11	0.570	0.154	
Pre-Rx	0.587	0.163	1.938
Rx 11	0.570	0.154	

TABLE 14-6
Differences in average total pausetime (SEC.)

Source	Mean	SD	t
Pre-Rx	0.081	0.098	-9.34*
Rx 1	0.480	0.267	
Rx 1	0.480	0.267	3.30*
Rx 11	0.310	0.306	
Pre-Rx	0.081	0.098	-5.11*
Rx 11	0.310	0.306	

*p<.05, df = 39 (2-tailed)

TABLE 14-7
Differences in mean interword pausetime (SEC.) for high/low probability sentences at the three treatment intervals

Source	Mean	SD	t
HI (PRE)	0.076	0.102	0.60
LO (PRE)	0.972	0.119	
HI (1)	0.413	0.244	2.38*
LO (1)	0.597	0.232	
HI (111)	0.232	0.243	1.72*
LO (111)	0.378	0.269	

* .01<p<.05, df = 19 (2-tailed)

** .05<p<.10, df = 19 (2-tailed)

15

The Use of Visual Feedback to Enhance Prosodic Control in Dysarthria

Michael P. Caligiuri

Thomas Murry

INTRODUCTION

Traditional treatment of motor speech disorders associated with neuro-pathologies is based on three principles: structural modification, increased functionality, or newly learned compensatory behaviors. The structure of speech musculature can be improved by various postural adjustments or prosthetic devices. The functionality of speech can be improved through increased muscular strength, range of motion, and tonicity by a regimen of isometric or isotonic exercises focusing on various muscle groups of the speech apparatus. Finally, dysarthric patients have shown improved speech intelligibility through the use of proper phrasing, speaking rate, or pacing.

Recently, instrumental approaches to treatment of motor speech disorders have gained acceptance. Investigators have employed feedback systems to improve functionality in dysarthric patients by monitoring electromyographic activity of articulatory musculature (Booker, Rubrow and Coleman, 1969; Daniel and Guitar, 1978; and Netsell and Daniel, 1979), intraoral and subglottal air pressure (Netsell and Hixon, 1978; and Netsell and Daniel, 1979), nasal air flow (Collins, Rubrow, Rosenbeck, and Gracco, 1981) and speaking rate (Berry and Goshorn, 1979, 1982). General findings suggest that many dysarthric patients benefit from treatment programs that provide feedback to one or more of the anatomic subsystems within the speech mechanism.

Modification of prosodic variables such as articulatory timing, speaking rate, loudness, melody, and pause time has been the principal objective of dysarthria treatment in a number of studies. Rosenbek, Collins, and Wertz (1976) used delayed auditory feedback to modify articulation time in a group of ataxic and hypokinetic patients. Rosenbek and LaPointe (1978) outlined procedures for teaching control of timing patterns in dysarthria. Other investigators such as Yorkston and Beukelman (1981), Murry (in press), and Berry and Goshorn (1979, 1982) discuss the use of treatment methods to teach control of speaking rate in patients with ataxic dysarthria.

The work of Berry and Goshorn (1982) and others suggests that visual feedback may be an effective treatment technique to teach control over other prosodic features such as physical effort, word duration, and intensity. The purpose of this investigation was to determine the effectiveness of visual feedback compared with nonvisual feedback treatment. Articulatory precision, speaking rate, prosody, and overall severity were the four criteria upon which treatment efficacy was assessed.

METHODS

Subjects

Three subjects were treated in this investigation. They were diagnosed by a speech pathologist as having acquired dysarthria in the absence of aphasia or apraxia of speech. Subject 1 was a 75-year-old male with pseudobulbar dysarthria secondary to bilateral CVAs. He was six years post onset. His speech was characterized as having articulatory imprecision, reduced articulatory range, excessive rate, monoloudness, monopitch, and prosodic insufficiency. Subject 2 was a 59-year-old male with ataxic dysarthria secondary to a cerebellar infarct. He was 5 months post onset. His speech was characterized by slow rate, prolonged segments, excess and equal stress, and overly precise articulation with inappropriate pitch and loudness variability. Subject 3 was a 61-year-old male with mixed dysarthria secondary to a 34-year history of multiple sclerosis. His speech decline began one year previously and was primarily ataxic and characterized by highly variable pitch and temporal contours, slow labored articulation, strident voice quality, and reduced loudness variation.

Instrumentation

Figure 15-1 shows a photograph of the apparatus used in the present study. The subject was seated facing a 4-channel storage oscilloscope (Tektronix 5013N).

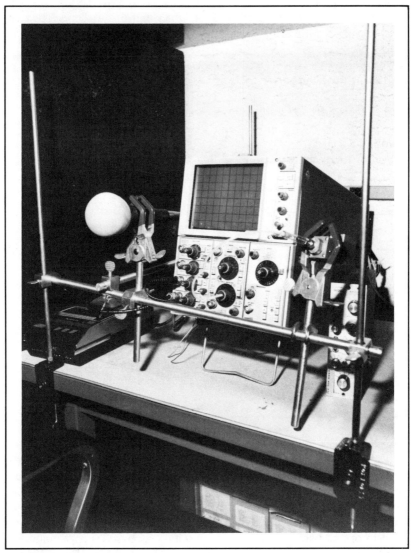

FIGURE 15-1
Apparatus used in this study

For the intensity and duration feedback phases, a microphone was positioned approximately 25 cm from the subject's mouth. For the intraoral air pressure feedback phase, a polyethylene tube was placed in the subject's mouth behind the point of articulation. The tube was attached to a differential pressure transducer (Statham PM 131) and a Honeywell bridge amplifier (Acudata 113). For all feedback phases, a modeled response was provided by the clinician and stored on the upper half of the scope. The subject's responses were displayed on the lower half of the scope.

Treatment Procedures

The recording and treatment phases are outlined in Table 15-1.

TABLE 15-1
Design of the treatment and recording sequence

WEEK	SESSION	DESCRIPTION
0	A	Recording
	B	Visual Feedback 1
3	A	Recording
	C	Visual Feedback 2
6	A	Recording
	D	Visual Feedback 3
9	A	Recording
	E	No-Treatment
12	A	Recording
	F	No-Visual Feedback
15	A	Recording

Four three-week treatment phases and one three-week no-treatment phase were provided for each subject. The first nine weeks consisted of three three-week periods in which visual feedback was provided to the subject about word duration, vocal intensity, and intraoral air pressure associated with target stress. The order of the three feedback phases was counterbalanced among the three subjects to allow analysis of treatment effects unrelated to order. Each treatment session within a phase lasted 40 minutes. There were six sessions per treatment phase. Visual feedback allowed the patient to monitor self-generated changes in intensity, duration, or intraoral air pressure of the stressed syllable or word. The no-treatment phase always preceded the final treatment phase. The final treatment phase did not employ visual feedback; rather, the clinician and patient relied upon the auditory modality to determine the accuracy of responses.

Stimuli

Table 15-2 shows examples of the stimulus items at seven levels of complexity. The stimuli used in treatment were created so that each target word or syllable contained a plosive consonant in the initial position. The number of items within each level ranged from 4 to 20.

TABLE 15-2
Examples of stimulus items and levels of complexity

LEVEL	STIMULUS TYPE	EXAMPLES
1	CV Nonsense Syllables	/pa/, /ba/, /da/, /ta/
2	CVC Meaningful Words	pan, boat, dime, toy
3	CVCVC Nonsense disyllables: Contrastive Stress	paPA, PApa, baBA, BAba
4	CVCVC Meaningful Words	Dodger, Teacher, Badger
5	3-Word Phrases: Contrastive Stress	PASS the peas. pass the PEAS.
6	Sentences: Contrastive Stress	Dave's DAD met his date, Dave's dad met his DATE.
7	Sentences Varying with Pragmatic Intent	Bob bought the box. vs Bob bought the box?

The same stimuli were used for all treatment phases and were administered in the following progression: CVC nonsense syllables, CVC words, CVCVC nonsense disyllables, CVCVC words, three-word phrases, five to seven-word sentences, and sentences varying in pragmatic intent. For levels having items of greater than one syllable, a contrastive stress paradigm was used to teach prosodic control.

Analyses

Six speech samples (that is, pretreatment, four interim treatment, and post-treatment audio recordings) were obtained from each subject (refer to Table 15-1). At each recording, a subject read the Grandfather Passage (Darley, Aronson, and Brown, 1975), one of the six 50-word Modified Rhyme Test lists (House, Williams, Hecker, and Kryter, 1965) and a list of 15 phrases of a contrastive stress drill. The Grandfather Passage and contrastive stress drill samples were used in the present study to assess treatment efficacy.

The sentence "Except in the winter when the snow or ice prevents, he slowly takes a short walk in the open air each day" was extracted from the Grandfather Passage. This sentence was paired with one taken from the other five recordings, totaling 15 different pairs. In addition, five of the pairs were repeated to assess listener reliability. The 20 sentence pairs for each subject were duplicated 4 times for presentation to listeners. The listeners were instructed to select the more normal of each pair based on their judgment of articulatory precision, speaking rate, prosody, and severity. Pre- and post-treatment samples were assigned a percentage score corresponding to the number of reliable listeners selecting that sample as more normal. Listeners were said to be reliable if for a given perceptual category they achieved a score of 75% or greater based on a test-retest method.

Analysis of the phrases spoken by the three subjects served as the basis for the second measure of treatment efficacy. Three trained listeners were instructed to select the cue or cues to word stress they perceived each subject used. Response choices included pitch, intensity, duration, or combinations of the three. There were pre- and post-treatment samples, each consisting of 15 phrases. Percentage scores, corresponding to the frequency of usage for pitch, duration, and intensity were obtained from the listeners based on agreement of 2 out of 3 listeners.

RESULTS

Perceptual Judgments

The results obtained from reliable listeners for the four perceptual categories of articulatory precision, speaking rate, prosody, and overall severity were used to compare the effects ascribed to visual feedback and nonvisual feedback. The reliability scores for the 13 listeners were generally low, and the number of listeners reaching criterion reliability (75%) ranged from 2 to 9 depending on the perceptual category.

TABLE 15-3
Percentage of listeners judging improvement over baseline for three subjects for four perceptual categories following visual feedback and no-visual feedback prosodic treatment

Subject	VISUAL FEEDBACK				NO-VISUAL FEEDBACK			
	Articulatory Precision	Speaking Rate	Prosody	Severity	Articulatory Precision	Speaking Rate	Prosody	Severity
1	25	78	50	25	0	22	50	0
2	0	33	100	50	75	22	50	50
3	75	78	100	100	100	22	100	100
Number of Listeners	4	9	2	4	4	9	2	4
Mean Reliability:	75%	75%	84%	81%	75%	75%	84%	81%

Table 15-3 shows how the listeners rated the post-treatment samples for each of the four categories for each subject. Percentage scores greater than 50% shown on this and subsequent tables demonstrate that more than half of the listeners judged the post-treatment sample as the more normal one. Each subject performed differently under the two treatment conditions. For the visual feedback, subjects 1 and 2 showed improvement in one category each, while subject 3 was judged to be more normal for the post-treatment sample in all four categories. For the non-visual feedback condition, subject 1 was not judged improved in any of the four categories. Subject 2 was judged improved in one and subject 3 was judged improved in three categories. These data are graphically described in Figures 15-2 through 15-5.

FIGURE 15-2

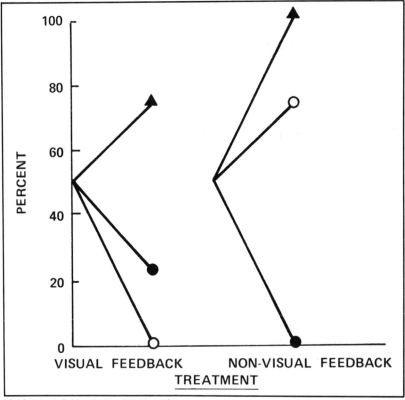

*Subject 1 (•), Subject 2 (0) and Subject 3(x)

Percentage of listeners selecting the post-treatment sample from two treatment conditions as more normal in articulatory precision for the three subjects.

Figure 15-2 shows the percentage of listeners selecting post-treatment as improving articulatory precision for the three subjects. The figure shows that visual feedback resulted in improvement for subject 3 only, whereas the no-visual feedback treatment resulted in improved articulatory precision for subjects 2 and 3. Figure 15-3 shows the percentage of listeners selecting post-treatment as improving speaking rate for the three subjects.

FIGURE 15-3

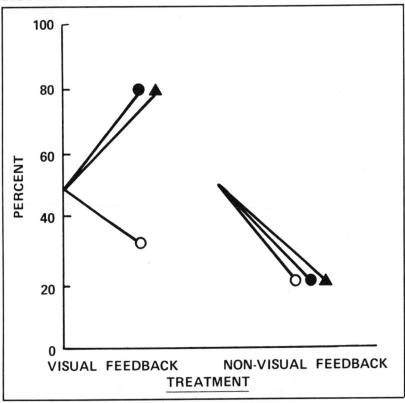

*Subject 1 (•), Subject 2 (0) and Subject 3(▲)

Percentage of listeners selecting the post-treatment sample from two treatment conditions as more normal in speaking rate for the three subjects.

Visual feedback resulting in improved speaking rate for subjects 1 and 3, whereas the no-visual feedback treatment did not improve speaking rate of any subject. Figure 15-4 shows the percentage of listeners selecting post-treatment as improving prosody for the three subjects. Again, visual feed-

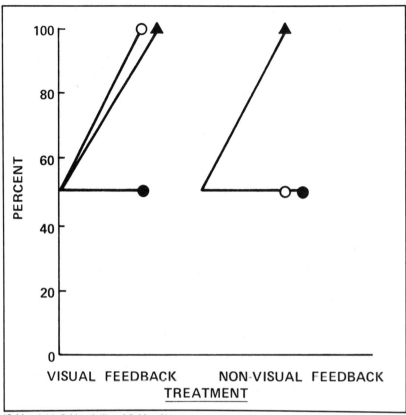

FIGURE 15-4
Percentage of listeners selecting the post-treatment sample from two treatment conditions as more normal in prosody for the three subjects.

back resulted in improvement for two subjects while the no-visual feedback condition resulted in improved prosody for one subject only. Figure 15-5 shows the percentage of listeners selecting post-treatment as improving overall severity. Only subject 3 demonstrated improvement in overall severity following both treatment conditions.

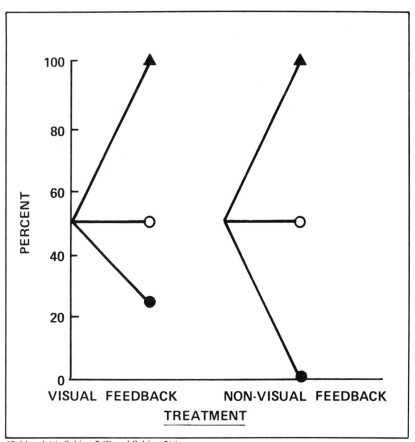

*Subject 1 (•), Subject 2 (0) and Subject 3(▲)

FIGURE 15-5
Percentage of listeners selecting the post-treatment sample from two treatment conditions as less severe for the three subjects.

While post-visual-feedback-treatment-percentage values were based on combined effects of three methods, the individual contributions of visual feedback of intraoral air pressure, duration, and intensity were found to be highly variable from subject to subject. Table 15-4 shows the analysis of listener responses to post-treatment effects for the perceptual category or categories under which improvement was shown for each subject. Subject 1

TABLE 15-4
Analysis of listener responses to post-treatment effects for three subjects
for the improved perceptual category and corresponding treatment week.

Subject	Improved Perceptual Category	Treatment Method	Weeks in Treatment
1	Speaking Rate	Pressure	3
2	Prosody	Intensity	9
3	Articulatory Precision	Duration	9
	Speaking Rate	Pressure	12
	Prosody	Duration	9
	Severity	Pressure	12

improved in speaking rate following intraoral air pressure feedback which occurred during the first three weeks of treatment. Subject 2 improved in prosodic control after the administration of intensity feedback during the sixth through ninth week of treatment. Subject 3 improved in two categories after duration and intraoral air pressure feedback were administered. Administration of these phases of treatment occurred during the sixth through twelfth week of treatment.

From Table 15-4 we can see that intraoral air pressure feedback was the most responsible for improvement, duration somewhat less, and intensity only improved ratings of normalcy in one perceptual category in one subject. Table 15-4 also reveals that those feedback conditions which demonstrated improvement were generally toward the end of the nine-week visual feedback program. Only once did a treatment method result in improvement after three weeks; that was the case for intraoral air pressure for subject 1.

Use of Perceptual Cues to Word Stress

The results obtained by three listeners identifying acoustic cues to word stress are shown in Table 15-5. It can be seen that each subject performed differently for the two treatment conditions. Subject 1 demonstrated a 20% increase in the use of duration following 9 weeks of visual feedback prosodic treatment. Subject 2 demonstrated a 20% increase in the duration following the no-visual feedback treatment. Subject 3 did not demonstrate an increase in the use of any of the rated perceptual cues to word stress following visual feedback; however, he did demonstrate a 27% increase in the use of pitch intensity following the no-visual feedback treatment.

TABLE 15-5
Percent change from baseline for three subjects in usage of pitch, intensity, and duration as perceptual cues to word stress following visual feedback and no-visual feedback prosodic treatment.

	VISUAL FEEDBACK			NO-VISUAL FEEDBACK		
Subject	Pitch	Intensity	Duration	Pitch	Intensity	Duration
1	0	− 20	+ 20	+ 13	+ 14	+ 40
2	− 20	− 46	+ 20	− 13	− 13	+ 34
3	− 7	− 20	− 60	+ 27	+ 27	− 14

DISCUSSION

The results of this study have shown that feedback-based prosodic treatment contributed to improved ratings of normal speech for three dysarthric subjects. Specifically, nine weeks of visual feedback resulting in improvements in speaking rate, prosodic control, and a reduction in overall severity. Since the aim of this study was to modify some prosodic features associated with speed production, it is not surprising that the changes in speaking rate and prosody were greater than that of articulatory precision. Improvement in articulatory precision, as demonstrated by subject 3, may reflect generalized gains associated with speaking rate and prosodic control. The finding that nonvisual feedback prosodic treatment resulted in improved articulatory precision for two subjects might be explained on the basis that the subjects received nine weeks of treatment prior to beginning the nonfeedback phase. Therefore, improvement in articulatory precision may reflect the influence of time in treatment rather than the type of treatment.

While no attempt was made to combine the visually based feedback with the more auditorily based treatment, it is likely that the benefit of auditory monitoring was present throughout all of the treatments, visual as well as nonvisual feedback.

Based on the perceptual ratings, subjects improved primarily after intraoral air pressure feedback and after nine weeks of any combination of visual feedback methods. Most gains in speed production were observed when comparing the pretreatment ratings with the ratings following nine weeks of treatment. This suggests that time in treatment played an important role in improving the speech of our subjects. Other studies have demonstrated that improvement in speech production may depend on the length of the treatment program. Berry and Goshorn (1979, 1982) were able to demonstrate the efficacy of visual feedback in improving speaking rate following 10 sessions. Of the 2 subjects studied by Collins et al. (1981), the subject who received 16 treatments improved in ratings of speech intelligibility; the subject with 9 treatments showed no improvements.

The perceptual ratings indicated a number of speech aspects were rated below the 50 percent level following treatment. Several factors must be considered before drawing conlcusions based solely on the use or effect of feedback. First, almost all analyses of subject 1 suggest a regression over time. His neurological and psychological status decreased over the course of treatment. His cognitive and perceptual abilities worsened and his family reported an increase in manic-depressive moments. These declines have been observed periodically throughout the six years since onset of his CVAs and probably contributed significantly to his regressive performance. Second, the methods of perceptual analyses may have been too stringent. Despite the selection of clinician-listeners familiar with dysarthria, their overall reliability was low, suggesting that their task was difficult. Previous research of treatment efficacy in dysarthria used a more general rating scale (Berry and Goshorn, 1979, 1982; Collins et al., 1981) to assess post-treatment changes. Furthermore, the first assessment of treatment efficacy was based on a sample taken from a spoken paragraph. Since treatment stimuli never reached complexity levels above a seven-word sentence, this assessment may not be indicative of improvements that occurred at levels of less complex stimuli. Finally, it was believed that the lack of change in speech production following the first phase of treatment for all subjects could be attributed to the small number of sessions, since each phase consisted of no more than six sessions.

The results of this study support the efficacy of visual feedback-based prosodic treatment in bringing about more normal speaking rate, prosodic control, and reducing overall severity in some dysarthric patients. Subtle changes in the way dysarthric patients utilize loudness, duration, or intraoral air pressure to impart syllable and word stress, which may go unnoticed without the aid of visual feedback, can be objectively measured. Visual feedback allows the clinician to observe a patient's strengths and weaknesses early in treatment. For example, subject 2 demonstrated no benefit from duration feedback; however, it appeared that he was able to benefit by using vocal intensity feedback.

Rubrow (1980) noted that while feedback systems have traditionally focused on events occurring early in the speech chain (e.g. electromyography), it is not known how effective a feedback system can be when it provides information to the talker about events occurring later in the chain (e.g. acoustic signal). This study supports previous investigations of feedback control which indicate improved speech production following treatment (Berry and Goshorn, 1979, 1982; Collins et al., 1981; Netsell and Hixon, 1978). Prosody, an integral part of the speech disorder associated with dysarthria, may also be addressed via the use of visual feedback. It is incumbent upon future investigators to determine the interrelationships of various feedback media, duration of treatment, and subject selection most responsive to this approach of prosodic control in the treatment of the dysarthrias.

REFERENCES

Berry, W., & Goshorn, E. Oscilloscopic feedback in the treatment of ataxic dysarthria. Paper presented to the American Speech-Hearing-Language Convention, Atlanta, 1979.

Berry, W., & Goshorn, E. A single subject design to assess the use of immediate visual feedback in the treatment of ataxic dysarthria. In W. Berry (Ed.), *Clinical dysarthria*. San Diego: College-Hill Press, 1983.

Booker, H., Rubrow, R., & Coleman, P. Simplified feedback in neuromuscular retraining: An automated approach using electromyographic signals. *Archives of Physical Medicine and Rehabilitation*, 1969, *50*, 621-125.

Collins, M., Rubrow, R., Rosenbeck, J., & Gracco, V. An instrumental approach to reduction of nasal emission in dysarthria. Paper presented to the American Speech-Language Hearing Association convention, Los Angeles, 1981.

Daniel, B., & Guitar, B. EMG biofeedback and recovery of facial and speech gestures following neural anastomosis. *Journal of Speech and Hearing Disorders*, 1978, *43*, 9-20.

Darley, F., Aronson, A., & Brown, J. *Motor speech disorders*. Philadelphia: Saunders & Co., 1975.

House, A., Williams, C., Hecker, H., & Kryter, K. Articulation testing methods: Consonantal differentiation with a closed-response set. *Journal of the Acoustical Society of America*, 1965, *37*, 158-166.

Murry, T. Treatment of ataxic dysarthria. In W. Perkins (Ed.), *Current therapy of communication disorders*. New York: Thieme-Stratton, in press.

Netsell, R. Evaluation of velopharyngeal function in dysarthria. *Journal of Speech and Hearing Disorders*, 1963, *34*, 113-122.

Netsell, R., & Daniel, B. Dysarthria in adults: Physiologic approach to rehabilitation. *Archives of Physical Medicine and Rehabilitation*, 1979, *60*, 502-508.

Netsell, R., & Hixon, T. A noninasive method for clinically estimating subglottal air pressure. *Journal of Speech and Hearing Disorders, 1978, 43*, 326-330.

Rosenbeck, J., Collins, M., & Wertz, R. Delayed auditory feedback in the treatment of dysarthric adults. Paper presented to the American Speech-Language-Hearing Association convention, Houston, November, 1976.

Rosenbek, J., & LaPointe, L. The dysarthrias: Description, diagnosis, and treatment. In D. Johns (Ed.), *Clinical management of neurogenic communicative disorders*. Boston: Little, Brown & Co., 1978.

Rubrow, R. Biofeedback in the treatment of speech disorders. In *SMCL Reprints*, University of Wisconsin, 1980.

Yorkston, K., & Beukelman, D. Ataxis dysarthria: Treatment sequences based on intelligibility and prosodic considerations. *Journal of Speech and Hearing Disorders*, 1981, *46*, 398-404.

ACKNOWLEDGEMENT

This study was supported by the Veteran's Administration.

16

Acoustic Analysis of Ataxic Dysarthria: An Approach to Monitoring Treatment

Nina N. Simmons

In recent years, there have been advances in the assessment and diagnosis of dysarthria. Darley, Aronson, and Brown (1969a and b, 1975) have contributed a perceptual system for differential diagnosis of type of dysarthria, and Yorkston and Buekelman (1981a and b) have given clinicians a more reliable means of measuring dysarthric speech intelligibility. However, objective measurement of prosodic or qualitative changes in speech remains a problem for most clinicians. Traditional approaches to evaluating prosody utilize rather general descriptors such as "monotone, scanning speech, lacking falling inflection." Other approaches such as relative stress ranking or stressing strategy questionnaires (Yorkston and Beukelman, 1980) help in analyzing prosody and planning treatment. However, they may not satisfy the demand for data based clinical accountability. Kent, Netsell, and Abbs (1979) proposed using acoustic analysis, demonstrating that sonographic recordings provided an objective measure of acoustic properties of ataxic speech, and suggesting that this might be a reliable means of documenting speech changes due to treatment.

To evaluate the usefulness of sonographic analysis in monitoring treatment effects, an ataxic patient undergoing speech therapy was studied.

METHOD

Case Presentation

H.Y., a 26-year-old man, sustained a closed head injury in a motorcycle accident, resulting in severe ataxia. He was first seen in our clinic seven years post onset. While language and memory were intact, speech was typical of ataxic dysarthria with excess and equal stress, slowed rate, monoloudness, and monopitch. H.Y. stated that after his accident he was seen briefly for speech therapy where he was instructed to "speak more slowly to avoid slurring his words." At the time we saw him, imprecise articulation was no longer a primary problem, but H.Y. felt (and we agreed) that he "sounded like a computer"; therefore, he was scheduled for speech therapy two hours per week to improve prosody.

Treatment

The program was divided into baseline and treatment periods. The baseline period involved audiotaping conversation and a reading of the "Rainbow Passage" over three consecutive sessions. Treatment phases were designed to improve prosody. Since prosody involves a complex interaction of speech behaviors, it was felt that separating target behaviors would simplify training. Therefore, treatment consisted of four phases.

For each phase a hierarchy of tasks was used to increase proficiency of the target behavior, while systematically increasing length and formulation demands. Responses were scored as target behavior present, target behavior absent, or target behavior partially present or distorted. Online scoring proved difficult; therefore, whenever possible, several dimensions were scored for each response. A level of 90% presence or partial presence was the criterion for moving from task to task in the hierarchy. Feedback included verbal explanation and audiotape replays. Stimuli, consisting of syllables, words, phrases, sentences, and paragraphs were changed from task to task.

Treatment Phase one (T1) involved training loudness and pitch variation (intonation), in order to reduce the monotone quality of H.Y.'s speech. After four months, 90% proficiency in varying pitch and loudness was achieved on the terminal task of reading a paragraph aloud.

At this point Treatment Phase two (T2) was initiated with emphasis on altering word and sentence stress patterns. H.Y. was taught to recognize stressed versus unstressed syllables and to vary production by inserting pauses prior to stressed units, lengthening stressed syllables, shortening unstressed syllables, and decreasing loudness or unstressed syllables. When stable performance for stressed/unstressed relationships was reached on reading a paragraph, treatment was shifted to Phase 3.

Treatment Phase three (T3) was designed to shorten syllable durations overall (ideally, while maintaining stress patterns). This included "corrupting" H.Y.'s articulation by slighting some consonants, underarticulating endings, and decreasing vowel durations.

As therapy progressed, it became apparent that training had actually produced new behaviors which diminished the naturalness of H.Y.'s speech; therefore, Phase 4 (T4) was aimed at decreasing exaggerated pitch and loudness variations, reducing the clipped, choppy quality caused by shortening words, and smoothing out transitions from word to word. This phase was completed approximately one year after initiation of baseline.

Acoustic Analysis

At the end of each treatment, phase audiorecordings of readings of the "Rainbow Passage" were made. Readings of this passage by two normal speakers were also recorded for purposes of comparison. After all phases of treatment were completed, selected portions of these recordings were subjected to analysis on a sound spectrograph. The utterance "when the sunlight strikes" was analyzed for baseline, each treatment phase, and normal subject using wide and narrow band recordings on a Key Elemetrics Model 7030A sonograph and a Series 700, VII Voice Identification Sound Spectrograph. Specific areas of interest on spectrograms included overall frequency contours, relative intensity of segments, pause time, and articulation time. Word boundaries were measured to determine duration in milliseconds, and spectrographic patterns of phonemes were compared to representations in Borden and Harris (1980) to ascertain any gross deviations from the expected.

Additionally, an analysis was made of three productions of "the rainbow" for the baseline and each treatment phase to determine the degree of H.Y.'s speech variability within each phase. Formant patterns showed no marked changes within each phase, and variability in duration was considered minimal (coefficient of variability ranged from .01 to .05).

RESULTS AND DISCUSSION

Analysis of the spectrograms proved quite interesting. As expected, H.Y.'s pretreatment (baseline) spectrogram showed a flat fundamental frequency contour (Figure 16-1). Positions of vowel formants appeared

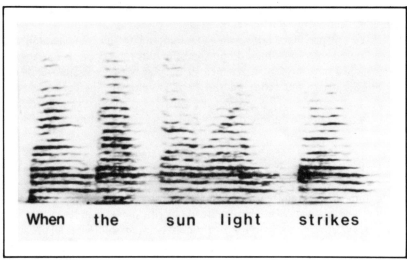

FIGURE 16-1
Narrow-band spectrogram for H.Y. at baseline

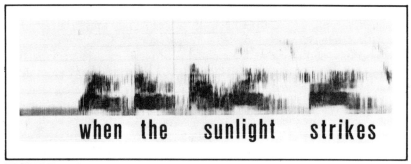

FIGURE 16-2
Wide-band spectrogram for H.Y. at baseline

normal, although there was a noticeable lack of high frequency energy (Figure 16-2). Osthoff (1979) suggested that a similar dissipation of upper formant energy among Parkinson's patients contributed to a flat, monotone quality. Perception of H.Y.'s speech as monotone and unnatural was probably attributable to the frequency contour and this energy distribution. The perceived "excess and equal stress" was represented on the spectrogram as essentially equal syllable durations with no variation in pause time for the phrase "when the sun light." Also, syllable durations were consistently longer than normal (Figure 16-3); the overall articulation time for H.Y. was 2438 msec. as compared to a mean of 1795 msec. for the normals.

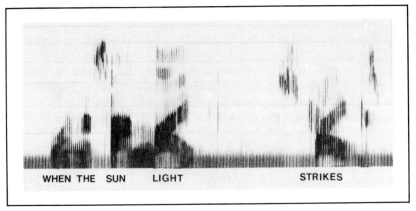

FIGURE 16-3
Wide-band spectrogram for a normal speaker

The spectrogram produced after the first treatment phase was surprising (Figure 16-4). Although treatment had focused entirely on pitch and loudness, the most striking changes occurred in the "time" dimension. The overall duration of the analyzed utterance markedly increased (from 2438 msec. to 3643 msec.), syllables were lengthened, and pauses were inserted. It is probable that H.Y. needed this extra time to produce the required pitch and loudness variations, but the resulting spectrogram looked even more deviant than the pretreatment one.

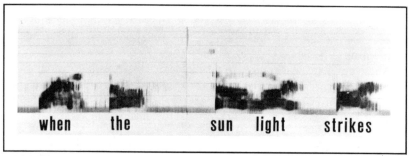

FIGURE 16-4
Wide-band spectrogram for H.Y. after Treatment phase 1

After the second treatment phase aimed at stress patterns, the proportion of time spent on each segment changed slightly, reflecting some variation in articulation time and pause time, but, again, the major change was an overall increase in duration (from 3643 msec. to 4153 msec.) (Figure 16-5).

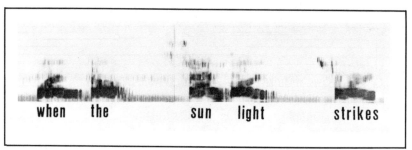

FIGURE 16-5
Wide-band spectrogram for H.Y. after Treatment phase 2

Also, decrease in the amount of "fill" and better definition of segment boundaries was noted; no doubt the inordinate amount of time allowed H.Y. to achieve better valving and more precise articulation.

The third phase of treatment attempted to decrease durations of syllables in general. The spectrogram showed overall duration decreased (from 4153 msec. to 3370 msec.) while retaining some variation in time spent on stressed and unstressed words (Figure 16-6).

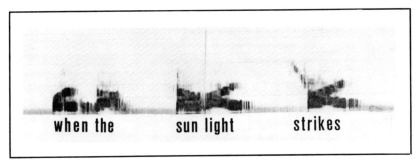

FIGURE 16-6
Wide-band spectrogram for H.Y. after Treatment phase 3

After Phase Four, the overall duration further decreased, the proportion of time spent on unstressed words decreased, and pauses were less exaggerated. The spectrogram (Figure 16-7) did not look like a normal speaker.

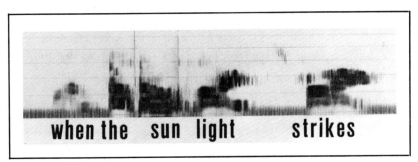

FIGURE 16-7
Wide-band spectrogram for H.Y. after Treatment phase 4

The overrall duration (2588 msec.) not only exceeded that of the normal speakers (Figure 16-3), but also exceeded that of the baseline recording (Figure 16-2) (2438 msec.); however, the pattern reflected more variation with less equalization of time.

Figure 16-8 schematically represents the durational changes in H.Y.'s speech over the source of therapy as compared to two normal speakers.

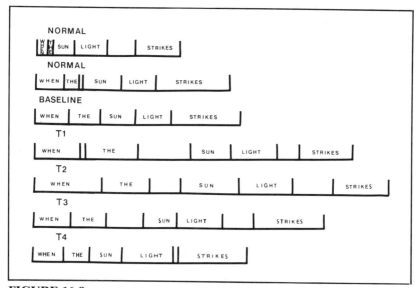

FIGURE 16-8
Schematic representation of relative pause and articulation times on production of the phrase "when the sunlight strikes" by 2 normal speakers and 5 samples of H.Y.'s speech

Syllable durations for normal speakers and each sample of H.Y.'s speech are shown in Figure 16-9. It is obvious from these data that durational elements were an important consideration during treatment (even when therapy did not specifically target this as in Phase 1). Analysis of these spectrograms suggested that target behaviors were not independent; working on specific aspects of speech, such as intonation or pitch variation, caused changes in other areas, such as time and articulation. As H.Y.'s scores on specific tasks were improving, other aspects of prosody were deteriorating. Monitoring effects of treatment with spectrographic analysis has the potential to pinpoint these interrelated effects and improve the efficiency of our treatment programs.

In the final analysis, H.Y. did show improved scores on tasks designed to improve prosody. He showed objective changes in acoustic properties on the spectrograms; however, H.Y.'s speech did not approach normal. It appeared to get farther acoustically from normal before it got better, and overall time actually increased in the final product. Obviously the goal, as in all dysarthria therapy, was compensated speech rather than normal speech; and a "trade off" of speech properties was made in an effort to make speech "sound better." Such an analysis of acoustic changes should help set goals, design treatment, and monitor progress as long as the clinician is aware of certain issues affecting interpretation and use of acoustic instrumentation.

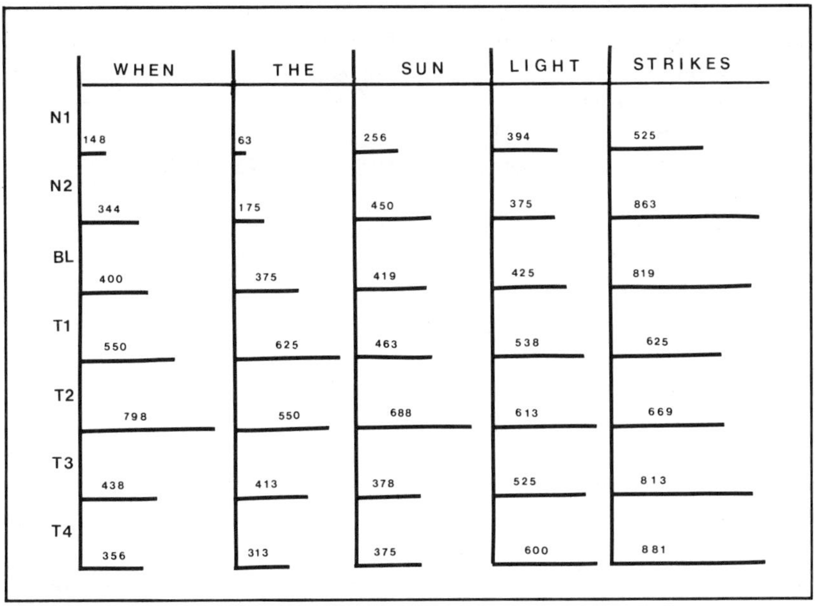

FIGURE 16-9
Comparative representation of articulation time in milli- seconds of each word of the phrase "when the sunlight strikes" for 2 normal speakers and 5 samples of H.Y.'s speech

All too often, clinicians avoid instrumentation as the sole realm of the speech scientist, anxiously proclaiming it to be too time-consuming, complicated, or research oriented. In fact, spectrographic analysis takes less time than scoring and analyzing many speech and language tests. The equipment is relatively easy to learn and use; the manuals give explicit step-by-step instructions, and information is available on interpretation of results (Painter, 1979). While there are many more accurate and sophisticated methods of evaluating speech acoustics, the sound spectrograph is one of the least expensive and most widely available systems.

The spectrogram can be placed in a patient's chart for objective documentation. It represents multiple parameters to assist in extracting interacting variables (this is very difficult to do by perceptual analysis) and serves as an excellent guide to improve the clinician's understanding of what the patient is doing to produce disturbed speech. Recordings of normal speakers can be made, and the literature contains considerable information on normal speech acoustics for purposes of comparison (Potter, Kopp, and Green, 1947; Borden and Harris, 1980). Spectrography is useful in measuring changes in speech due to treatment, surgery (Johns and Salyer, 1978) or progression of disease (Logemann, Fisher, and Boshes, 1972). It can be impressive evidence for physicians. In the continuing struggle to prove efficacy and accountability, the spectrogram is often viewed by others as more objective and scientific than descriptive information. This strengthens referral channels and enhances our position in the battle for funding.

It should be noted, however, that there is little information to help judge what constitutes "progress" on a spectrogram. We observe significant changes in certain parameters, but the judgment of how it sounds to the listener remains the ultimate measure of improvement. Clinicians must be aware that acoustic events do not translate directly to perceptual dimensions. Acoustic analysis is not a substitute for listening, it simply adds to our understanding of what we perceive. Both types of analysis contain subjectivity in interpretation. Our expectations and labels can lead to erroneous assumptions. For instance, the clinician should realize that "pause time" as measured on H.Y.'s spectrograms simply represents absence of recorded speech sound; preparatory posturing, inspiration, imploding of air, or any number of activities may be occurring during this time. A similar problem occurs when noise appears on the spectrogram; it is the clinician's judgment whether this represents hypernasality, air escapage, or a poor recording. Dynamic or variable characteristics may be missed on short samples (usually 2.2 seconds per spectrogram). Therefore, the clinician's choice of utterances analyzed is extremely important.

Measurements taken from the spectrogram (voice onset time, formant frequencies, etc.) may vary, causing questionable reliability. When comparing successive spectrograms on one patient, consistency in measurement is important. If results are to be compared to published measures, or across clinicians, agreement of several clinicians is needed. Variables involved in audiorecording must be controlled to eliminate artifacts such as intensity changes due to varying the distance from the microphone, intrusion of background noise, etc.

Another limitation of spectrographic analysis is the lack of immediate feedback for the patient and clinician. The ideal situation is instrumentation combining immediate feedback, hard copy printouts, and recording of multiple parameters on line. Not only is this technology available, but it is also conceivable that hospitals and clinics will eventually hook into central computers where voice samples will be fed in routinely for immediate acoustic evaluation. The present reality is that the sound spectrograph is available in many clinics. Therefore, speech clinicians should explore sound spectrography as a clinical tool. Decisions on the usefulness of acoustic analysis should be based on clinical applications and awareness of limitations and strengths. Not only is further study of this area likely to improve interpretation of treatment results, but it will also help us understand what is happening in therapy, and how we can make it happen more efficiently.

REFERENCES

Borden,G., & Harris,K. *Speech Science Primer*. Baltimore: Williams & Wilkins, 1980.

Darley,F., Aronson,A., & Brown,J. Clusters of deviant speech dimensions in the dysarthrias. *Journal of Speech and Hearing Research*, 1969, *12*, 462-496. (a)

Darley,F., Aronson,A., & Brown,J. Differential diagnostic pattern of dysarthria. *Journal of Speech and Hearing Research*, 1969, *12*, 246-269. (b)

Johns,D., & Salyer,K. Surgical and prosthetic management of neurogenic speech disorders. In D. Johns (Ed.), *Clinical management of neurogenic communicative disorders*. Boston: Little, Brown and Co., 1978.

Kent,R., Netsell,R., & Abbs,J. Acoustic characteristics of dysarthria associated with cerebellar disease. *Journal of Speech and Hearing Research*, 1979, *22*, 627-648.

Logemann,J., Fisher,H., & Boshes,B. Frequency and progression of speech and voice disintegration in Parkinson's disease. *Trans. Am. Neuro. Assoc.*, 1972, *97, 301-03.*

Osthoff, D. Spectrographic analysis of hypokinetic dysarthric speech in Parkinson's disease. Unpublished research project. University of Kansas, 1979.

Painter,C. *An Introduction to Instrumental Phonetics*. Baltimore/ Univ. Park Press, 1979.

Potter,R., Kopp,G., & Green,H. *Visible speech*. New York: D. Van Nostrand Co., 1947.

Yorkston,K., & Beukelman,D. *Assessment of intelligibility of dysarthric speech.* Tigard, OR: C.C. Publications, 1981. (a)

Yorkston,K., & Beukelman,D. Ataxic dysarthria: Treatment sequences based on intelligibility and prosodic considerations. *Journal of Speech and Hearing Disorders*, 1981, *46*, 398-404. (b)

Yorkston,K., & Beukelman,D. Intelligibility and prosody as overall measures of dysarthric speech. Miniseminar presented at the American Speech-Language-Hearing Association convention, Detroit, 1980.

ACKNOWLEDGEMENT

The author wishes to acknowledge Dr. McKay Burton, New Orleans VAMC, and Dr. Donald Rampp, LSU Medical Center, Department of Audiology & Speech Pathology for generously allowing the use of acoustic analysis instrumentation.

17

Special Considerations for the Development of Microcomputer-Based Augmentative Communication Systems

Craig W. Linebaugh
James T. Baird
C. Bruce Baird
Richard M. Armour

An attitudinal shift in favor of functional communicative competence and the introduction of increasingly sophisticated augmentative communication systems (ACS) have been among the more prominent recent trends in the management of dysarthric individuals. The relationship between these two trends is necessarily symbiotic. As we, as clinicians, and the communicators whom we serve place greater value on communicative success, regardless of the means by which it is achieved, we all more readily invest our resources in developing and using ACS. Not that we forsake speech, but that communication holds the premier position among our objectives. Reciprocally, advances in ACS application and technology, particularly as they enhance communicative efficiency, free us to pursue the goal of functional communicative competence more aggressively, while at the same time making "augmented communication" more acceptable to our patients.

The purpose of this chapter is to discuss a number of considerations with which clinicians should be familiar as a new wave of ACS breaks over us. This wave consists of ACS which have at their hub a microcomputer. Already, a substantial number of such systems are in use (IEEE Computer Society, 1981), and with the continued rapid development of microcomputers, they will likely become the systems of choice. In this chapter we are seeking to prepare the clinician to confront this new wave—to provide a basic awareness of the inherent advantages and potential of such systems, and the difficulties which might be confronted.

SPECIAL CONSIDERATIONS: ADVANTAGES

Communication Needs

The range of communicative situations in which the patient may need to adequately and efficiently express himself must be carefully analyzed. Two factors in this analysis are the mode and permanence of output. Depending on the patient's requirements, transient graphic, permanent graphic, or speech output can be employed, singly or in combination.

The types of utterances the patient needs to produce both routinely and in critical, though infrequent, stituations should also be considered. The memory capacity of a microcomputer permits storage of longer utterances or sequences of utterances than do most conventional electronic devices, thus allowing more information to be conveyed more readily. High priority utterances can be stored so that they may be retrieved in the most expedient manner. In addition, programs can be utilized which enable the user to add or delete specific utterances to or from the memory in accord with his changing needs.

Communicative Efficiency

Perhaps the single most important factor with regard to the eventual acceptance and use of an ACS by a patient is the efficiency or speed with which he can communicate. A system employing a microcomputer can incorporate several features not generally available in other types of devices. This is especially true for patients requiring a scanning selection mode. First, a hierarchical message access structure can be employed. Rather than using a scroll-type display or a single, static matrix or menu, a microcomputer can provide a sequence of matrices. Beginning with a master or control matrix, the patient can call up secondary matrices, tertiary matrices, and so on. The hierarchy or matrices or menus can be organized according to topic, need, or any other convenient organization scheme. Figure 17-1 depicts one possible format for a hierarchical message access structure.

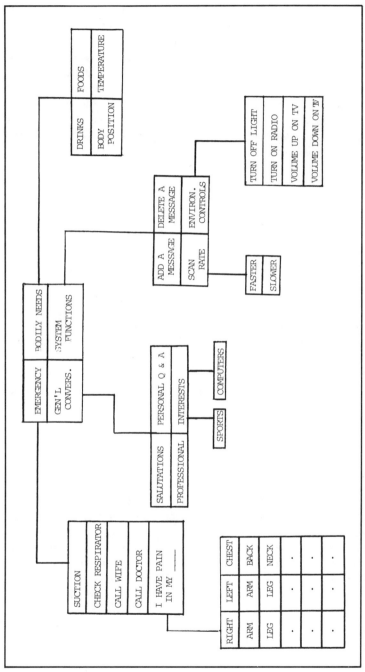

FIGURE 17-1: A sample hierarchical message access structure.

Second, the microcomputer can be programmed to reorder the matrices or menus by frequency of use after a predetermined number of selections. In so doing, however, certain priority constraints should be observed so that emergency entries remain highly accessible. Third, the scan rate (dwell time) can be continually adjusted to the patient's level of performance by the computer. This can be accomplished by an increase or decrease in the scan rate based on a fixed select:backspace (error) ratio or the user's consistently responding in designated portions of the dwell time. A special self-calibration program can also be used to set the initial rate or to adjust the rate at appropriate intervals.

Cognitive-Linguistic Abilities

The inherent capabilities of today's microcomputers are such that the needs of cognitively and linguistically sophisticated users can be readily met. Judicious organization of the computer's memory and use of encoding strategies can permit such individuals to produce lengthy, complex utterances with considerably greater efficiency than they could by other means.

Moving along the user continuum toward those with limited cognitive or linguistic abilities, the computer offers the means of providing compensatory adjustments. For those with limited reading ability, computer-generated pictographic displays can be used. One system is currently available which employs blissymbols (The Talking Blissapple, Trace Center, 1981). Programs are also available which facilitate word retrieval (Colby, Christinaz, Parkinson, Graham, and Karpe, 1981) and the use of various syntactic forms (Hillinger, 1981). The computer-based ACS can, therefore, provide the user with a display appropriate to his cognitive and linguistic level, and produce a normalized graphic and/or speech output.

Medical Status

The patient's medical status is another factor for which the microcomputer has special applications. For the patient whose condition is stable, the repertoire of utterances and applications is limited only by the memory capacity of the computer and the patient's ability to utilize it. The greater advantage, however, accrues to the patient whose condition is fluctuating or progressively deteriorating. For the patient with fluctuating attention, strength, reaction time, etc., a calibration routine can be employed to adjust scan rate to the patient's condition at a particular time. For the patient whose condition is deteriorating, the computer can be used to accumulate data on various efficiency parameters (e.g., backspace, scanning through the display without making a selection), and, at appropriate times, system upgrades can be implemented to meet the patient's changing needs.

Severity of Limb Involvement

A microcomputer-based system is especially applicable to the patient with severe limb involvement. Not only can such systems operate on virtually any type of switching input, they can also provide a computer-assisted direct selection mode utilizing various types of analog input. We have developed one such system utilizing electromyographic activity. Another, using eye movements, was developed by Mark Friedman of Carnegie-Mellon University and his colleagues (Friedman, 1981). Regardless of the input mode, the assessments of activation force, range and resolution of motion, reaction time, and replicability of response as need be made in determining an appropriate interface for other devices (Coleman, Cook, and Meyers, 1980) similarly apply to computer-based systems. An additional advantage of the computer-based system, however, is that it can be programmed in a manner to enhance the resolution of less than optimal motor responses.

Visual Acuity

Compensations for patients who experience difficulty seeing a standard CRT display because of decreased visual acuity can be accomplished using the graphic capabilities available with many microcomputers. Larger than standard-sized letters, symbols, or figures can be generated, and color contrasts utilized, where beneficial. For those with severe visual impairments, including blindness, speech output can be provided as the selections are scanned.

Training

The effective use of any ACS requires training, and computer-based systems offer a unique advantage in this regard. A training protocol can be provided to help the user learn the most efficient ways of operating the system. Instructions can be displayed where useful. "Games" of various types can be used to help the patient improve his reaction time and resolution and replicability of response. Programs can also be developed to aid in the learning of specific commands and retrieval codes. Likewise, special programs can be developed to facilitate the learning of phonetics for systems requiring phonemic encoding to produce novel utterances in speech output, or the "modified" spelling required to achieve optimal intelligibility with certain "text-to-speech" devices (e.g., Type-'N-Talk by Votrax).

The patient must also learn to place the transfer of information above grammatical or spelling perfection. This is essential if the individual is to achieve the most efficient communication possible with a particular system. Recent enhancements in programs for computer-based systems, however, have diminished the need to sacrifice grammatical form in favor of communicative efficiency. Of note is the program developed by Hillinger (1981), which permits the production of various syntactic forms from a minimal number of entries.

Support

Use of any ACS requires some level of support from family members and others involved in the patient's care. This is particularly true of some electronic devices. While a computer-based system does require a relatively high level of support during its development, once the system is in place, this need is limited essentially to "start up" and "housekeeping" routines. In addition, equipping the system with various environmental control devices reduces the severely-involved patient's level of dependence in other areas.

Educational / Vocational / Recreational

The educational potential of microcomputers is only beginning to be tapped, and the benefits which may accrue to severely-handicapped individuals, who might otherwise experience even greater limitations in their educational opportunities, are enormous. A computer-based system can also be employed in a patient's vocational rehabilitation and, possibly, in the performance of certain job-related tasks apart from communication. In addition, the recreational potential of a microcomputer is extensive, and offers an important outlet for the patient who is unable to participate in other forms of recreation. All of these applications can contribute significantly to the individual's self-esteem and psychological well-being.

SPECIAL CONSIDERATIONS: DISADVANTAGES

Listener Reactions

Because the patient needs to focus his attention on the display while formulating his messages, he is, in essence, isolated from the nonverbal reactions of his listeners during these periods. Chief among these reactions may be indications of impatience with the rate at which messages are developed, particularly if the patient persists in correcting inconsequential errors or producing unnecessarily elaborate responses. There is a delicate balance between the user's desire to produce "normal" utterances and his listener's desire to "keep the conversation flowing." This requires training and counseling for all those routinely involved with the system.

Portability/Security

Until recently, portability represented a limiting factor in the provision of computer-based ACS. The combined weight of computer, display, power supply, and keyboard, or switch, required the use of some sort of cart to transport the system. This was acceptable for the nonambulatory patient, but markedly restricted the potential use of such systems by the ambulatory. Now, however, the continued miniaturization of microcomputers has brought us to the threshold of being able to provide ambulatory patients with a highly portable system with both speech and graphic output.

An issue related to portability is that of security. Larger systems requiring a cart are inherently less vulnerable than more portable systems, but must occasionally be left exposed when the user enters a place inaccessible to the cart. Conversely, the more portable system, which the user can keep with him at all times, is more readily removed by those who would do so. Regrettably, as microcomputers become an ever more desirable product, they become a more likely target of theft. As a result, the security of the system should be considered from the inception of its design.

Cost

The cost of the hardware required for a microcomputer-based ACS is highly variable depending on the capabilities deemed necessary and desirable by the user. In most instances, however, an acceptable system can be assembled for approximately the same cost as other popular electronic communication devices which are more limited in their applications. Substantial cost can be encountered, however, in the course of software development. The more elegant and diverse the capabilities of the system, the greater will be the cost of developing the programs to carry them out. On the other hand, an acceptably efficient and flexible program utilizing a scanning selection mode with graphic output is commercially available for approximately $100 (Smith, 1981), and, reportedly, several others will soon become available at a reasonable cost.

THE FUTURE

When an individual is using an ACS to communicate, it is desirable that the system virtually disappear. That is, the communication between the user and his listeners should be as natural and intimate as that between two un-impaired speakers. While this may represent an unobtainable ideal, there remain to be made many strides in its direction. These strides need to be made along at least three paths.

The first path is in the area of hardware development. The continued placing of greater capability in smaller packages holds forth ever-increasing possibilities for refining ACS. The second area is that of software develop-ment. Further refinements need to be made to make systems more flexible and efficient in order that their users can attain "normal" speeds of infor-mation transfer in all modalities. The third, and most important area, is that of ergonomics, or human factors. It is in this area that speech-language pathologists can potentially make their greatest contribution in the contin-ued refinement of computer-based ACS. The physiological, perceptual, cognitive, linguistic, and emotional aspects of using ACS must be more clearly understood. The individual user's capabilities and reactions must be more effectively assessed and the system developed accordingly. With in-creased sophistication in developing computer-based ACS to meet the needs of individual users, the *interface* between the user and the ACS, and that between the ACS and the listeners, will become less prominent, and the *interaction* between the user and his listeners will be enhanced.

REFERENCES

Colby, K., Christinaz, D., Parkinson, R., Graham, S., & Karpe, C. A word-finding computer program with a dynamic lexical-semantic memory for patients with anomia using an intelligent speech prosthesis. *Brain and Language,* 1981, *14*, 272-281.

Coleman, C., Cook, A., & Meyers, L. Assessing non-oral clients for assis-tive communication devices. *Journal of Speech and Hearing Disorders,* 1980, *45*, 515-526.

Friedman, M. In *Proceedings of the Johns Hopkins First National Search for Applications of Personal Computing to Aid the Handicapped.* Los Angeles: IEEE Computer Society, 1981.

Hillinger, M. Computer-enhanced communication systems. In *Proceedings of the Johns Hopkins first national search for applications of personal computing to aid the handicapped.* Los Angeles: IEEE Computer Society, 1981.

IEEE Computer Society, *Proceedings of the Johns Hopkins first national search for applications of personal computing to aid the handicapped.* Los Angeles, 1981.

Smith, B., *Handicapped typewriter.* Vancouver, B.C.: Rocky Mountain Software, 1981.

The Talking Blissapple. Trace Center. In *Proceedings of the Johns Hopkins first national search for applications of personal computing to aid the handicapped.* Los Angeles: IEEE Computer Society, 1981.

Subject Index